HANDBOOK OF
PEDIATRIC
OPHTHALMOLOGY

Jean M Wright

HANDBOOK OF PEDIATRIC OPHTHALMOLOGY

Editors

Stephen S. Feman, M.D.
*Associate Professor
and Director of Retinal Services
Department of Ophthalmology
Vanderbilt University
Nashville, Tennessee*

Robert D. Reinecke, M.D.
*Professor and Chairman
Department of Ophthalmology
Albany Medical College
Albany, New York*

Grune & Stratton
A Subsidiary of Harcourt Brace Jovanovich, Publishers
New York   San Francisco   London

LIBRARY OF CONGRESS

CATALOG CARD NO.: 78-71861

Feman, Stephen S. and Robert D. Reinecke
Handbook of Pediatric Ophthalmology.

New York, N.Y.: Grune & Stratton
200 p.
7812   780905

Grune & Stratton, Inc.
111 Fifth Avenue
New York, New York 10003

Distributed in the United Kingdom by
Academic Press, Inc. (London) Ltd.
24/28 Oval Road, London NW 1

Library of Congress Catalog Number 78-71861
International Standard Book Number 0-8089-1115-5

Printed in the United States of America

Contents

Preface

As the medical specialties have become more fully developed and the sub specialties have become better defined, the volume of information involved has rapidly enlarged. This phenomenon has caused the production of encyclopedic textbooks in all fields. The reader can easily get lost in the morass of technical material. This handbook is intended to supply the reader with a broad overview and a basic understanding of the field of pediatric ophthalmology. It is our hope that this will facilitate more detailed pursuit of selected topics. Most of the references are to textbooks that describe each of these subjects in elaborate detail. Thus the reader can progress to any subject that is of specific interest and can study it in depth.

The authors would like to thank the third-year students at Albany Medical College, as well as our colleagues and friends. Their numerous questions and their requests for abbreviated crib-side consultations led us to an awareness that a "field guide" to children's eyes was needed. Gratitude must also be expressed to the many members of the faculty at the Albany Medical College who aided in the production of various portions of this book. In addition, we are most grateful to our wives, Edith and Mary, for their understanding and patience.

Stephen S. Feman, M.D.
Robert D. Reinecke, M.D.

List of Contributors

Stephen S. Feman, M.D.
Associate Professor and Director of Retinal Services
Department of Ophthalmology
Vanderbilt University
Nashville, Tennessee

John Griffin, M.D.
Assistant Professor of Ophthalmology
Albany Medical College
Albany, New York

Pei-Fei Lee, M.D.
Associate Professor of Ophthalmology
Albany Medical College
Albany, New York

Ian Porter, M.D.
Professor of Pediatrics
Albany Medical College
Albany, New York
and Director, Birth Defects Institute
State of New York

Robert D. Reinecke, M.D.
Professor and Chairman, Department of Ophthalmology
Albany Medical College
Albany, New York

Richard S. Smith, M.D.
Professor of Ophthalmology
Albany Medical College
Albany, New York

HANDBOOK OF
PEDIATRIC
OPHTHALMOLOGY

Robert D. Reinecke, M.D.

1
Vision, Amblyopia, and Strabismus

The purpose of this chapter is to suggest an orderly approach in dealing with children suspected of having visual defects or misaligned eyes. In any such examination vision must be a primary concern, and only by notations of impressions of visual status can appropriate referral or reassurance be accomplished. In general, if a visual defect is suspected, the earlier it is investigated the better is the potential for successful therapy.

A brief review of what constitutes visual acuity should serve as an appropriate background. Visual acuity (normally a test for central vision) is the ability to detect two lines separated by a space equal to the width of the line. This is called minimum separable acuity and is the type of acuity used in the construction of all visual acuity charts. Obviously this is considerably different from minimal detectable acuity, which can be likened to the ability to see a white spot on a dark background or a star in the sky. Such types of acuity testing are difficult to use, although occasionally they must be employed. Examples of such instances include having a child follow a rolling marble on the floor or follow a moving flashlight. Obviously, we are testing rather crude visual acuity when we resort to such determinations. As each age group is considered, the most appropriate visual acuity test will be mentioned.

NEWBORNS

To make a successful visual examination of a newborn, it is necessary that the child be in a receptive mood, that is, awake but not crying or feeding. Awakening a newborn from sleep prevents any estimation of visual acuity. A newborn who is awake and receptive should easily be able to follow the movement of the examiner's face above the crib. As a flashlight is brought from either side, the child will tend to look toward the light. Moving objects are more attractive to the child than stationary objects. Since one of the principal objectives of all vision testing is to determine the visual ability in each eye independently, it is necessary to use some means of covering each eye sequentially. This does not mean that a hand must be put close to the child's face; interception of the pupillary axis is all that is necessary. Occasionally, a hand can be held over one eye at close range, but in most cases occlusion at a considerable distance from the eye will be less threatening to the child. Before doing that, it is a good idea to assess (as far as possible) the ability of the child to look about. Then one should carefully occlude each eye without disturbing the child, taking note of any change in the reaction. Most children will tolerate this quite well because they can see equally well with either eye. If a change in performance is detected as one eye is covered, this should be interpreted as poor visual acuity, and further tests are in order.

When there is difficulty in covering the eyes, it is appropriate to have a nurse place an adhesive patch over one eye prior to the arrival of the examiner in the nursery. The nonoccluded eye should be checked on that particular visit; if necessary, the opposite eye can be occluded during a similar sleeping period so that the other eye can be tested on the next visit to the nursery.

The use of small test objects is, of course, inappropriate, since it is impossible for a child to respond in any fashion other than simply to seek out a flashlight or wiggling fingers. The optokinetic drum is occasionally useful, since if the child does have detectable optokinetic nystagmus (see Chapter 6), use of the drum will confirm that the child has vision in that eye. Since most optokinetic drums have extremely large stripes, this confirms no more than crude vision.

The next step is to look into each eye to determine if the child will fixate with the fovea. This is easy to do with newborns if they are examined at the appropriate time. The direct ophthalmoscope is used with the aperture reduced so that a small circle of light is all that the child and the examiner can see. By looking into the child's eye from very close range, the examiner will be able to see the foveal area. Usually the child will cooperate, and the disk can be examined as well. Children of this age are usually extremely cooperative; there is no excuse for not examining the fundus in detail. Should any questions remain concerning the child's vision, the pupils should be dilated for a complete examination.

The quality of the foveal reflex is not good in any child, and one must be careful not to equate an absence of shiny foveal reflex with poor visual acuity. The foveal area is slightly granular, and the entire fundus typically will have a blond appearance in most children. Even in a black child the fundus will be remarkably pale, as compared to fundi in black adults.

In the newborn child who has nystagmus, it is well to note carefully any instability of fixation as well as transillumination of the iris. One should not be alarmed by the amplitude of the nystagmus; typically, it will decrease with time. It should also be noted that the newborn's optokinetic nystagmus may be rather poor in quality. Overconcern with this poor response should not lead the examiner into reporting poor vision to the parents.

If iris transillumination is present, complete albinism may be diagnosed. Ocular albinism can be difficult to detect at birth, since typically the iris does not transilluminate. As the child is followed along, by 6–10 years of age the iris will begin to transilluminate in a detectable fashion. Ocular albinism, which may be incomplete as far as lack of pigment is concerned, shows slightly reduced visual acuity, but most such children will do relatively well in the long run.

Newborns may have misaligned eyes (strabismus). The eyes may turn in, out, or up. Any type of misalignment should cause concern to the examiner, for it may indicate poor vision in one eye at that time or that amblyopia is developing secondary to the strabismus. Although it is true that in rare instances children will have misaligned eyes that subsequently will become straight, in most instances this is a myth, it should be quickly dispelled in favor of the more reasonable deduction that the child is likely to have permanent strabismus. Hence it is important that vision in these children be followed carefully to be certain that an amblyopia is not developing.

In conclusion, the newborn who has misaligned eyes is a real cause for concern, and the child who does not see well with each eye should be suspected of having a serious problem.

CHILDREN 3 MONTHS TO 1 YEAR OF AGE

Children 3 months to 1 year of age are more difficult to examine than newborns, but the same parameters are applicable. By this time it is usually easier to determine whether or not strabismus is present. By far the most helpful feature is whether or not some member of the family has detected a turned eye. If the parents report that the eye is turned in, but the examiner is unable to detect esotropia (by alternately covering one eye at a time and noting whether or not the eye has to move out to pick up fixation), the concern is probably not valid. On the other hand, if the parents report that the eyes turn out, but examination does not confirm exotropia, it is best for the examiner to believe the parents and proceed on the basis that the child does have intermittent exotropia. Any serious suspicion of a misaligned eye should once again trigger a careful follow-up to be sure that amblyopia does not develop. Certain tests have been developed (e.g., the use of smaller and smaller marbles rolled across a dark carpet) to assay the amount of vision in this age group. Most of these tests are not very satisfactory; clinical impression of the child's perfor-mance as each eye is occluded is a much better assay. Should the examiner have further concern, it is appropriate to give the parents some adhesive eye patches and have them cover one eye at a time (for an hour or so) to observe the child's performance. The child should perform the same with either eye covered.

CHILDREN 1–2.5 YEARS OF AGE

During the period from 1 year to 2.5 years of age strabismus, should it develop, is most likely to be noted. Hence, careful strabismus history from the parents is quite important. The previous notations in regard to parents' history are applicable in this age group. It is tempting to try "illiterate E" testing, Landolt ring testing, and other specific visual acuity tests during this period of time. Generally these are unsuccessful, and it may be best not to burden the routine examination with such attempts. It is better to be certain that the eyes are aligned, which may be done by alternately occluding each eye and deter-mining any refixation movement, and similarly noting whether or not the child has difficulty in performance with either eye covered. Should any strabismus be detected, it is essential that the child be followed carefully to ensure appropriate refractions and glasses (if necessary), appropriate patching for amblyopia, and surgery should other methods fail to align the eyes. Data have shown that early approaches to misaligned eyes give much better long-term effects.

CHILDREN 2.5–4.5 YEARS OF AGE

Children 2.5–4.5 years of age generally cooperate sufficiently well in the office that visual acuity testing in a conventional manner may be carried out if sufficient effort is made. However, a screening test is more appropriate. For the pediatrician's office, the screening test we recommend is that for stereop-sis. Although it does not allow determination of visual acuity in the usual sense, a high level of stereopsis confirms good and equal vision. There are a number of tests available, but generally the random-dot E test is by far the best. Polaroid glasses are placed in front of the child, and three cards are used to determine the stereopsis. Since there are no other clues available that allow the random-dot E cards to give false readings of good stereopsis, the test has an appropriate referral rate and is very successful. Instructions come with the test and need not be detailed here.[1,2]

In the event that such a test is not available, one must employ the visual acuity tests in the usual fashion. Kits of figures measurable to 20/30 called Allen figures are helpful in this early age group. Unfortunately, the tumbling

E blocks and picture cards give what is known as isolated visual acuity, i.e., looking at an isolated letter as opposed to a full line of print. Isolated visual acuity is typically better than linear acuity; indeed, it may mask amblyopia. Hence, care must be taken in interpreting isolated visual acuity as being equal to full-line visual acuity.

It may be helpful at this point to review briefly what is meant by the Snellen equation. For practical reasons the Snellen eye charts are constructed so that *each detail* (i.e., each line and each space between two lines) of the letter or figure on the 20/20 line will subtend a 1-minute angle when viewed at 20 feet. The notation 20/20 means that a distance of 20 feet the eye can resolve a target the size of which subtends an angle equal to a total height of 5 minutes of arc. Most adults with normal eyes achieve this 20/20 vision. The notation 20/30 means that letters that subtend a total arc of 5 minutes at a distance of 30 feet can be visualized at only 20 feet. When the distance is 20 feet but the height of the letter is that which a 5-minute arc would subtend at 200 feet, the designation is written 20/200. Conversion to the metric scale is easy because 6/6 (meters) equals 20/20 (feet). Hence, 6/12 would equal 20/40. Many times the testing distance in the examiner's office will be shorter than the distance required for the standard acuity chart. Thus, if there is a 20/20 line, but it is viewed at 10 feet, that should be noted as 10/20; it is, of course, equivalent to 20/40. If there is a 20/10 line on the visual acuity chart and it is measured at 10 feet, then this should be recorded as 10/10, which is equivalent to 20/20.

Many children are remarkably advanced in knowledge of the alphabet by virtue of watching many hours of television. Hence, it is appropriate to try the standard Snellen acuity chart before resorting to any other test, other than the stereopsis screening test. If at all possible, the complete line should be used for testing, rather than isolated letters. It is also important, of course, to carefully occlude each eye independently as vision is tested. Appropriate eye treatment too often is delayed because the child has peeked from under a cover during vision testing. Every effort should be made to avoid that pitfall.

The concerns previously mentioned in determining visual acuity also apply to alignment of the child's eyes. If the eyes are not aligned, further investigation into the possible cause is extremely important. One cannot emphasize the cardinal rule too often that the earlier strabismus and amblyopia are treated, the better the result.

CHILDREN 4.5 YEARS OF AGE AND OLDER

Testing visual acuity in children 4.5 years of age and older is usually the same as testing an adult. Charts that have full lines of letters should be used. Careful notation of the testing distance should be made, and the same attention should be given to preventing the child from peeking out from under the cover during the testing period. The stereopsis screening test is equally valid for all age groups and is particularly appropriate for the preschooler, since it is easily and quickly administered.

If poor vision is detected, referral is usually the logical course; however, should the presence of pathology be a concern, use of the pinhole effect is one of the handiest means of differentiating organic from refractive visual problems. Defective vision, if optical in origin, will be corrected by use of the pinhole. Hence, simple visual acuity measurements done monocularly and then again with a pinhole will confirm whether the poor visual acuity is due to some organic defect or is due simply to the need for an optical correction. It is often helpful to show myopic children how to simulate a pinhole (by curling the index finger into a small tunnel) so that those who lose their gasses can see to get about.

We may summarize visual acuity and strabismus testing as follows: Always look for the fixation response to be certain that the eye is capable of seeing. Whenever possible, use visual acuity test targets that are measurable, with careful notation as to the distance they are held from the patient. Any discrepancy from one eye to the other should be cause for referral. Above all, do not succumb to the myth that eyes will straighten if given sufficient time. Turned eyes mean that a problem exists, and appropriate attention should be given immeditaely.

STRABISMUS

There are several types of strabismus and various etiological factors involved, this section will attempt to outline some of the common ones.[3]

Esotropia

Esotropia (crossed eyes) is one of the more common problems in children. Indeed, about 3–4 percent of patients will have esotropia of some variety. From a screening point of view, this is an exceptionally rewarding area to cover. Some children will have esophoria rather than an esotropia. In esophoria there is a tendency for the eyes to turn in, but the child is able to straighten the eyes when given the opportunity. If the child is tested carefully, the tendency to turn in can be noted. As the cover is removed from one eye and the child is allowed to view things binocularly, the eyes will suddenly become straight. These children have a tendency to deteriorate from esophoria to esotropia. Thus, early attention should be given them whenever possible. Children who are extremely farsighted fall into a similar category. As they make an attempt to see objects clearly, the eye has to accommodate an exceptional amount, and the accommodative-convergence reflex turns the eyes in excessively. Hence, when the child is relaxed, the eye may be straight, but when the child attempts to look carefully at an object, *intermittent esotropia* will be noted.

Since one of the basic determinations in esotropia is refractive error, as mentioned previously, and since the eyes often can be straightened with glasses alone, accurate assessment of the optical defect is essential. This assay, high on the ophthalmologist's priority list, is accomplished by cycloplegic refraction.

Many ophthalmologists use atropine, and the dosage is rather high considering the size of the patient. Hence, it is not uncommon for a mildly toxic reaction to be reported by the parents. This toxic reaction will result in the child becoming febrile and having a flushed appearance with dilated pupils. This should not be confused with any illness. It is logical to inquire whether a child who is febrile has been to an ophthalmologist recently. The toxicity usually is not great; the best advice to the parents is to cease administration of the atropine and simply take the child's temperature at reasonable intervals. If no significant hyperthermia develops, then they should keep the next appointment with the ophthalmologist. In rare instances patients may develop hyperthermia or other significant side effects; then appropriate antidotes may be given.

More commonly used are the shorter-acting cycloplegic agents. They also may cause flushing of the skin and may even give rise to mild disorientation and drowsiness. The latter signs are usually seen in younger children or fair-complexioned children. Drowsiness typically lasts 2–3 hr. Hence, reassurance can be given about such children. Occasionally a patient will have a short convulsion, but treatment with barbiturates is seldom necessary.

Often the ophthalmologist may use an objective means of measuring the child's optical error. This is called retinoscopy and is quite precise, so that glasses may be prescribed for the child of any age, from a few days on.

Esotropia also may be caused by sixth nerve paralysis. Any time esotropia develops suddenly, concern regarding the numerous possibilities that can give rise to a defective sixth nerve should always be at the back of one's mind. Fortunately, lateral rectus paralysis secondary to sixth nerve interruption is not common, and in the majority of cases it may be self-limited. The reader is referred to Chapter 6 for further details.

A and V patterns are common in esotropia; these are descriptive terms related to the vertical position of greatest esotropia. The V pattern means that when the child looks down, the eyes become crossed; when the child looks up the eyes may be quite straight. Since most of the time when a person looks down the eyelids cover the eyes, esotropia in downgaze is not easily noted at an early age. As a result, these often are not detected until the child becomes older and someone is in a position to see the eyes in downgaze. Conversely, the child who has A esotropia has a greater crossing when looking up. In other positions of gaze, the eyes may be quite straight. Indeed, many of these children do not need treatment, but they may be a cause for concern to the parents until the children grow tall enough to look the parents straight in the eye.

One of the more interesting features of these patients with A and V patterns is the tendency of the oblique extraocular muscles to overact. When such a child looks to one side, the adducting eye (the eye looking toward the nose) may suddenly rotate up or down. The cosmetic effect may be traumatic to parents and child alike, but the implication is not important other than in the treatment of the A and V patterns.

Exotropia

Exotropia (walleye or turned-out eye) typically develops as a child gets older (i.e., 6–10 years of age) but it may present at any time, even in the neonatal period. The majority of these patients demonstrate an intermittent tendency that often is not noticeable until the child becomes older. One of the early symptoms the parents will report is that on going outside the child will close one eye. One reason for this is that in bright light the eyes have a tendency to turn out, and the exotropia becomes manifest; the child then closes one eye in order to avoid diplopia. Nearsightedness (myopia) is sometimes associated with the exotropia and will be suitably corrected on referral. The exotropia, because it is intermittent, allows development of good stereopsis at near vision; hence, the eyes work well together most of the time. Because of this, treatment for exotropia is not as aggressive from a surgical standpoint as is treatment for esotropia. An esotropic patient has a great tendency toward not using the two eyes toegher, whereas the exotropic patient does well in this regard, and surgery may be delayed until the exotropia becomes more constant. However, if exotropia is present in extremely young children, surgery often is indicated earlier, since these children will not have straight eyes for any significant time during a 24-hr period.

A and V patterns are noted among exotropic patients, with A patterns somewhat more common than V patterns (i.e., when the child looks down, the eyes may turn out to a greater extent). The overacting obliques also may be noted in exotropia; hence, the child looks rather bizarre when attempting to look to either side, when the adducting eye may turn up or down excessively.

Refractive Errors

Throughout the preceding discussion we mentioned the need for glasses and the essential nature of refraction in all patients with strabismus or amblyopia. One of the reasons for this is that the eyes may have different refractive errors; hence, the image in one eye may be blurred while the image in the opposite eye may be clear. The child tends to suppress this blurred image, causing amblyopia. Eyes may be nearsighted or farsighted or may have astigmatism. Astigmatism simply means that the cornea of the eye is shaped more like the surface of a lemon, as opposed to the usual spherical shape of most corneas. This irregularity can be easily corrected with appropriate spectacles.

A few words of explanation about refractive disorders may be helpful in explaining these problems to parents.[4]

Myopia or nearsightedness. A positive family history typically is present in the child who is found to be nearsighted. Often the parents are extremely concerned about the child having to wear nearsighted glasses, as they have had to do throughout their lives. Unfortunately, there is no means of prevention of nearsightedness, but parents should be reassured that the vision will be as good as theirs or perhaps better and that appropriate contact lenses can be prescribed any time that the child's age permits or the parents deem them appropriate. Whereas it is true that some forms of nearsightedness become so extreme that vision can be poor, the majority of patients will have good vision, and glasses are an appropriate solution to the problem. If the myopia is severe, yearly examinations are in order, since these large eyes are more susceptible to retinal detachments.

Farsightedness. The average child is farsighted at birth, and this gradually becomes less severe as the child's eye grows and becomes normal in size. Mention has already been made of the association between farsightedness and esotropia. Suffice it to say that whenever amblyopia or esotropia is suspected, the child obviously must be refracted; if hyperopia is present, that must be fully corrected. If the hyperopia is not severe or if bifocals are required, drugs may sometimes be used in place of glasses to control the excessive convergence that some of these patients manifest. This is termed a high accommodative-convergence/accommodation ratio. Miotics such as echothiophate iodide (Phospholine Iodide) may be used that cause miosis and cause the eye to react as if it has already accommodated; hence, it will not require as much accommodative convergence. Often these drugs are remarkably successful in controlling esotropia, thus avoiding the need for surgery. Since these are long-acting miotics, it is important to be aware that they can cause side effects, including gastrointestinal upsets. Anesthesia can be somewhat hazardous by prolonging the effect of succinylcholine if it is used. Thus it is mandatory that whenever anesthesia is advocated, inquiry be made as to whether or not the child has been receiving eyedrops.

Treatment of Amblyopia

In addition to the use of glasses to correct any refractive error, patching is the basis for all amblyopia treatment. The good eye is patched in such a way that the patient cannot peek out from under the patch. The patch must be worn all the waking hours, and many ophthalmologists prefer that the child wear the patch 24 hr per day. The child should return to the ophthalmologist's office at regular intervals, since prolonged occlusion can produce amblyopia of the eye that is being patched at the same time that the amblyopia of the opposite eye is being treated. Thus careful follow-up is essential. Many parents become discouraged during the occlusion therapy, and the child assumes control of the entire treatment. Reinforcement from the pediatrician is an extremely helpful feature during this period of time. It gives the parents hope that the treatment will eventually terminate, and it ensures that appropriate cooperation is elicited from the child as well. The patching may require as long as 1 year to complete, and it may have to be intermittent after that time. Thus it is a long-term problem, and no shortcuts are available.

Strabismus Surgery

Sooner or later many patients need surgery. The surgery is brief, and hospitalizations are not prolonged. Modern surgical treatment of strabismus includes the use of strong sutures with relatively atraumatic surgical techniques employed in such a fashion that the two eyes are never patched at the same time. Typically, the patient can go home either the same day of surgery or the following day. The child should be able to return to school within a few days after surgery.

It is important for the pediatrician and parents to realize that strabismus procedures may have to be repeated. Repeated surgery offers the same percentage of success as the original surgery. In general, failure of the eyes to be aligned after surgery, although disappointing to the parents and surgeon, must not be viewed with alarm. The surgery is of such a nature that it can be repeated several times without any danger to the eye. There are numerous surgical techniques that generally are effective either in weakening a muscle by moving its insertion farther back on the globe or in strengthening a muscle by moving its insertion forward on the globe or by removal of a short piece of the tendon or muscle. Even the latter (a resection) is not irreversible, since the muscle can simply be moved back a bit (recessed), or an additional piece can be resected from it.

As the child is being cleared for strabismus surgery, the pediatrician must be concerned that the child is in sufficiently good health to withstand 1.5 hr of anesthesia.

REFERENCES

1. Reinecke RD, Simons K: A new stereoscopic test for amblyopia screening. Am J Ophthalmol 78:714, 1974

2. Simons K., Reinecke RD: A reconsideration of amblyopia screening. Am J
    Ophthalmol 78:707, 1974
3. Reinecke RD, Miller D: Strabismus: A Programmed Text (ed 2). New York,
    Appleton-Century-Crofts, 1977
4. Reinecke RD, Herm RJ: Refraction: A Programmed Text (ed 2). New York,
    Appleton-Century-Crofts, 1976

Stephen S. Feman, M. D.

2

Children with Uncommon Appearances

The incidence of human congenital malformation is unknown. The major factors that influence such statistical data are related to the eagerness with which such features are searched for, as well as the methods of reporting and collating findings. Macroscopic physical congenital deformities are estimated to occur in 25 of every 100 live births.[1] Ocular abnormalities may have a greater incidence because they are less obvious and are not reported in a standardized manner. Some ophthalmic variations may represent isolated benign features in an individual, or they may be indicative of a syndrome involving multiple organ systems. The number of syndromes that have specific ophthalmic findings is quite large. The following disorders represent those seen most frequently in a general pediatric clinical environment.

STRUCTURAL ABNORMALITES OF THE SKULL

Stenotic Disorders

Stenotic disorders are the most frequent structural abnormalities that cause ocular changes. This is because of a premature closing of the skull sutures, or craniostenosis. In response to this stenosis, growth of the skull bones will be in other than normal directions, producing a misshapen skull. In addition, if the premature closure involves the orbital region, continued growth of the ocular tissue in the shallow orbit will produce exophthalmos.

A representative of the stenotic disorders is the acrocephalosyndactylia

13

of Apert, which is the most common systemic generalized osteodysplasia involving the orbit (Fig. 2-1). It is probably due to general mesodermal disturbance in the eighth week of embryogenesis. The prominent front-pointing skull is associated with fused and webbed fingers, as well as with other anomalies. The high-pointing frontal bones produce shallow orbits, exophthalmos, proptosis, maxillary hypoplasia, and dental defects. The systemic manifestations include synarthroses of multiple limb joints, polycystic kidneys, and uterine abnormalities.

Dysostotic Disorders

The dysototic disorders of ocular importance are those associated with embryologic defects of the branchial arches. One portion of the first branchial arch develops into the upper facial stuctures, and the other portion forms the lower facial structures. When the defect involves the maxillary segment of the first branchial arch, there can be defects of the eyelids and cheeks. This is noted in the dominantly inherited craniofacial dysostosis of Crouzon that is characterized by a front-bossing skull, maxillary hypoplasia, and a protruding prominent mandible. This maxillary defect is associated with shallow orbits, exotropia, and exophthalmos, and it permits many of these patients to voluntarily luxate their eyes anterior to the bony orbit (Fig. 2-2)

Defects of the mandibular portion of the first branchial arch are charac-

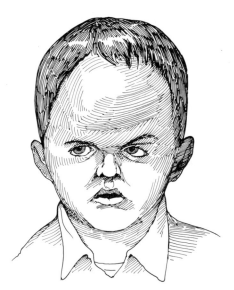

Figure 2-1.   Acrocephaly: high-pointing frontal bones and maxillary hypoplasia.

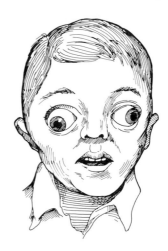

Figure 2-2. Craniofacial dysostosis: front-bossing skull, maxillary hypoplasia (shallow orbits, exotropia, exophthalmos), prominent mandible.

terized by a receding chin. The Treacher-Collins syndrome is a well-known example of this group of disorders. It is an association of hypoplasia of the lower jaw, a small mouth, malformed ears, and a nose that appears beaked and prominent when compared to the hypoplastic mandible.

Defects of the first and second branchial arches produce Goldenhar's syndrome. Patients with this problem have inferotemporal epibulbar dermoids, low-set ears with excessive auricular appendages, and vertebral anomalies.

DISORDERS OF THE CERVICAL VERTEBRAE

Patients with disorders of the cervical vertebrae give the appearance that the head is attached to the shoulders without any neck present. Such individuals have neurologic and skeletal defects. The Klippel-Feil syndrome is typical of this problem. The Klippel-Feil syndrome is a congenital synostosis of the upper cervical vertebrae. It appears as if the head is fused directly to the body. Platybasia and torticollis are noted commonly, as are defects of the cervical nerves. The extremities demonstrate mirrorlike movements that may be related to abnormalities of motor tract decussation. The eye findings are strabismus, external ophthalmoplegia, and nystagmus.

CUTANEOUS DISORDERS

Disorders of the skin of the lids and face are among the most common ocular problems. There are disorders that involve all of the skin but that are most noticeable in and around the eyes, whereas there are other disorders that involve only the ocular tissue. Albinism, in its various forms, can represent both types of disorder.

Systemic Albinism

Systemic albinism is a relatively common disorder with an incidence of 1 in 20,000 persons. There are at least two distinct varieties of systemic albinism; each is caused by a single specific enzyme defect in cellular metabolism of the amino acid tyrosine.[2]

The first type is associated with a defect in the permeation enzyme that transports tyrosine into the cell. The other enzymes within the cell that react with tyrosine, such as tyrosinase, are normal. Tyrosinase-positive albinism is associated with a blue or lightly pigmented iris, mild nystagmus, photophobia, and poor visual acuity that may improve with age.

The second kind of generalized albinism is caused by a deficiency of tyrosinase within the cell, Tyrosinase-negative albinism is associated with gray-blue irides, severe nystagmus, photophobia, and persistent visual loss.

Ocular Albinism

Ocular albinism is usually an X-chromosome-linked disorder. In the affected male the pigment deficiency is restricted to the ocular tissues. The skin and hair may be hypopigmented, but these tissues improve in time. The female carrier may have a characteristic clinical appearance. The ocular pigmentation may occur in scattered clumps at the level of the retinal pigment epithelium. This is believed to represent a clinical manifestation of the Lyon hypothesis; that is, in a female each cluster of cells is activated by a different X-chromosome.[3]

Ataxia-telangiectasia

Ataxia-telangiectasia (Louis-Bar syndrome) is an autosomal recessive disorder that includes an association of ataxia due to progressive cerebellar atrophy, oculocutaneous telangiectasia, and defects of the immune system. The cerebellar atrophy produces ataxia in the first 4 years. Telangiectasia of the face and conjunctiva are noted soon after the ataxia. An oculomotor disturbance is manifested by a defect of voluntary movement and a disturbance of conjugate gaze. Agammaglobulinemia or hypogammaglobulinemia permits the recurring infections that result in the death of these children. An increased incidence of malignancy has been reported.

Basal Cell Nevus Syndrome

Basal cell nevus syndrome patients have multiple cutaneous nevi in which basal cell carcinomas develop in the second decade. Most often the nevi are noted in the skin of the face and in the eyelids. Maxillary and mandibular cysts are associated with defective dentition. Vertebral anomalies and a wide variety of neurologic abnormalities have been reported in these patients. In addition, hypertelorism, strabismus, synophrys, and colobomas are noted frequently.[4] Visual acuity is within the normal range.

Cockayne's Syndrome

Cockayne's syndrome is a recessive disorder in which cutaneous, skeletal, and neurologic defects are noted in the first year. The facial skin is light-sensitive and develops an erythematous reaction; this results in an atrophic area of variegated pigmentation. The skeletal defects are dwarfism, microcephaly, and joint deformities. The neurologic manifestations include pigmentary retinal degeneration, optic atrophy, mental retardation, cerebral atrophy, and intracranial calcification.

DISORDERS ASSOCIATED WITH INBORN ERRORS OF METABOLISM

The most typical and most often seen inborn error of metabolism is the systemic albinism that was described earlier. However, so many of the inborn errors of metabolism have ocular manifestations that the other common syndromes need to be described.

Alkaptonuria

Alkaptonuria is a recessive disorder in which there is a deficiency of homogentisic acid oxidase. This enzyme is needed for the metabolism of phenylalanine and tyrosine. The excess homogentisic acid will be excreted in the urine, where it will produce a characteristic brown staining of diapers. The associated pigmentation of cartilagenous and collagenous structures is called ochronosis. This can produce darkly pigmented spots in the sclera as well as the cartilage of the ears and nose. These patients have good vision.

Homocystinuria

Homocystinuria is a deficiency in the cystathionine synthetase enzyme, and it has an autosomal recessive inheritance. This is among the most common metabolic defects in mentally retarded patients. The metabolic defect results in the excretion of homocystine in the urine, which facilitates the diagnosis. The elevated blood levels are associated with widespread vascular thromboses that may create a hazard during surgery. A prominent ophthalmic feature in these patients is dislocation of the lens into the anterior chamber, which produces secondary glaucoma; this may be precipitated by dilation of the pupil. The developing glaucoma may be the presenting symptom; the mental retardation and blotchy skin may not have been extreme enough to indicate this clinical diagnosis at an earlier time. Dietary management may offer substantial benefits to some of these patients.

Other disorders that may be classified as inborn errors of metabolism will be found in the section on mucopolysaccharidoses.

CHROMOSOMAL ABNORMALITIES

Disorders associated with chromosomal abnormalities are described in detail in several other chapters. For that reason, the following is a brief description of the disorders in children with uncommon appearances.[5]

Deletions of Chromosome 5

Deletions of chromosome 5 (Cri du chat syndrome) have been noted in children who have microcephaly and micrognathia in association with hypotonia, mental retardation, and the characteristic cry. Ocular findings include hypertelorism, epicanthal fold, and colobomas.

Defects of D Chromosomes

Defects of chromosomes of the D group are reported in children who have microcephaly and severe retardation. Their most common ocular features are hypertelorism, epicanthus, ptosis, microphthalmia, and colobomas. An unusually high incidence of retinoblastoma is reported in patients with a partial deletion of the Dq variety.

Trisomy 21

Trisomy 21 (Down's syndrome) is a common autosomal abnormality. These patients have mental retardation and hypotonia. Brachycephaly and stubby hands with a single palmar crease are characteristic findings. Epicanthal folds, Brushfield spots, and esotropia are noted in most cases (Fig. 2-3).

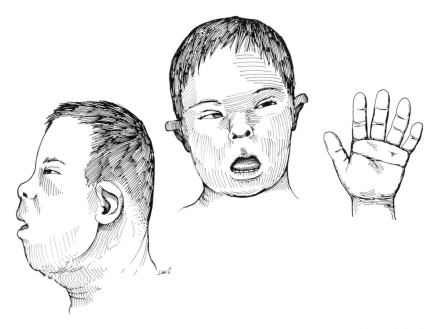

Figure 2-3.   Trisomy 21: brachycephaly, epicanthal folds, stubby hands, and single palmar crease.

Trisomy 13

Trisomy 13 (Patau's syndrome) is manifest by cleft lip and palate. Ocular abnormalities are the second most common feature in these patients. Microphthalmia and uveal colobomas are reported frequently in association with a wide variety of other ophthalmic anomalies.

MUCOPOLYSACCHARIDOSES

The mucopolysaccharidoses (MPS) are a group of disorders that involve many portions of the eye. A detailed table relating to all members of this group will be found in another chapter. The associated metabolic defects produce accumulations of mucopolysaccharides within body tissues and cause excretion of acid mucopolysaccharide into the urine. The clinical manifestations of these disorders are noted in some children with uncommon appearances; such patients have characteristic gargoylelike faces, skeletal defects, and varying degrees of connective tissue abnormalities, cloudy corneas, and retinal degeneration.[6]

Hurler's Syndrome

Hurler's syndrome (MPS-I) is an autosomal recessive defect in production of the enzyme iduronidase. This results in urinary secretion of dermatan sulfate and heparan sulfate and is associated with corneal clouding, retinal degeneration, mental retardation, and death from cardiac or pulmonary anomalies in the first decade of life (Fig. 2-4).

Scheie's Syndrome

Scheie's syndrome (MPS-V) is similar to Hurler's syndrome in regard to certain biochemical and hereditary features: dermatan sulfate is found in the urine, and recessive inheritance is noted. However, there must be some additional unknown feature in these children because their faces are not extremely abnormal, their intelligence is normal, and their life expectancy is not severely reduced.

Hunter's Syndrome

Hunter's syndrome (MPS-II) is biochemically similar to Hurler's syndrome, but Hunter's syndrome is an X-linked recessive disorder that features less severe systemic abnormalities, clear corneas, and longer life expectancy.

Sanfilippo's syndrome

Sanfilippo's syndrome (MPS-III) is an autosomal recessive disorder characterized by heparan sulfaturia. Several enzyme defects have been impli-

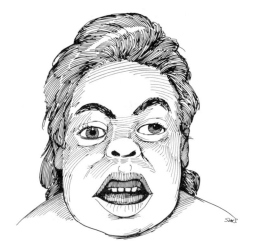

Figure 2-4.   Mucopolysaccharidosis, the characteristic appearance of Hurler's syndrome.

cated, but clinical patterns are similar. These patients have clear corneas and somatic defects less severe than those in Hurler's syndrome, but the mental deficiency is more pronounced.

Morquio's Syndrome

Morquio's syndrome (MPS-IV) is an autosomal recessive deficiency of a hexosamine sulfatase enzyme that results in keratan sulfaturia. In addition to corneal clouding, these patients have dwarfism and severe skeletal defects. The defects permit spinal cord injuries, paraplegia, and death.

Marteaux-Lamy Syndrome

Marteaux-Lamy syndrome (MPS-VI) is an autosomal recessive cause of dermatan sulfaturia. These patients have cloudy corneas, dwarfism, and normal intelligence. However, hydrocephalus develops in these children and results in neurologic changes and death.

PHAKOMATOSES

The phakomatoses constitute a group of congenital disorders that are related by the fact that they have multiple disseminated hamartomatous tumors involving several organ systems. In most cases dominant heredity is noted. Not all of the phakomatoses produce children with uncommon appearances. Those that are not relevant to this chapter will be described only briefly; more detailed information may be found in other portions of this book.

Von Hippel-Lindau Angiomatosis

The disorder of von Hippel and Lindau consists of angiomas of the retina and cerebellum. These children do not have uncommon appearances. Retinal angiomas are present in most of these patients, and they are present in both eyes in more than half. More than one-third of these patients have central nervous system symptoms from intracerebellar angiomas. The incidence of asymptomatic intracerebellar angiomata must be higher. For this reason, all patients with this disorder need detailed neurologic evaluation.

Sturge-Weber Syndrome

Another angiomatous syndrome is that of Sturge-Weber. Its most characteristic feature is a flat, venous, subcutaneous hemangioma in the area of the trigeminal nerve. It is associated with angiomas of the meninges and/or choroid. When the meninges are involved, there are neurological symptoms such as epilepsy and hemiplegia. When the choroid is involved, glaucoma may be present. Cutaneous vascular anomalies involving other areas of the body have been described in these patients (Fig. 2-5).

Bourneville's Disease

The tuberous sclerosis of Bourneville is a non-angiomatous phakomatosis. Within the eye, the astrocytic hamartomas look like mulberry nodules on the retina. Specialized angiofibromas appear in many cutaneous areas. This is the adenoma sebaceum that appears to be pigmented papules over the nose and cheeks. Various neurologic symptoms may be noted when the astrocytic hamartomas are present within the central nervous system.

Von Recklinghausen's Disorder

Von Recklinghausen's disorder consists of widely disseminated neurofibromatomas. Every patient with this disorder has scattered cutaneous pigmentation known as café au lait spots. Multiple plexiform neuromas may appear as subcutaneous tumors bulging out under the skin. Neurofibromas of the skin may be found as pedunculated tumors near the eyes. Ophthalmic manifestations may include small intraocular tumors, but most frequently this disorder is associated with tumors that involve the retrobulbar intraorbital tissue or the eyelids. The central nervous system may have similar tumors and may produce a variety of symptoms.

Wyburn-Mason Syndrome

The Wyburn-Mason syndrome is another vascular phakomatosis that is seldom associated with an uncommon appearance. These patients have ar-

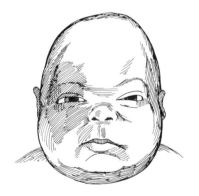

Figure 2-5. Encephalotrigeminal angiomatosis (Sturge-Weber): flat venous subcutaneous hemangioma in the area of trigeminal nerve distribution.

teriovenous malformations that appear as racemose angiomas of the retina and central nervous system. Rarely, an orbital hemangioma may produce proptosis.

ANIRIDIA

In aniridia a rudimentary iris is always present but is hidden beneath the corneoscleral border tissues. A detailed discussion of aniridia will be found in Chapter 3. However, certain characteristics warrant mention at this time. Dominant heredity is most common, but the recessive and sporadic cases are of great interest. As many as 20 percent of patients in the sporadic group may develop Wilms' tumor in the first 2 years of life.[7] Occasionally, Wilms' tumor has been reported in patients with the familial nonsporadic variety. Other renal abnormalities, such as horseshoe-shaped kidneys, often are noted in these patients with aniridia; therefore renal evaluation should be carried out for all such patients.

DISORDERS OF CONNECTIVE TISSUE

Connective tissue disorders can cause a patient to have an uncommon appearance. However, manifestations are not often noted in the pediatric age group. A few that present in the pediatric population have characteristic ocular findings.

Marfan's Syndrome

Marfan's syndrome is an autosomal dominant disorder characterized by long and thin extremities, dislocated lenses, and cardiovascular defects. A generalized defect of the elastic component of connective tissue is believed to be the primary abnormality. Typically, the lens dislocation is incomplete, bilaterally symmetric, and upward; cataracts and glaucoma can develop secondary to this problem. In most cases the long and thin extremities are associated with joint deformities and muscle hypoplasia. Congenital cardiac anomalies occur in more than one-third of these patients, and dissecting aortic aneurysm is a frequent cause of death.

Weill-Marchesani Syndrome

The Weill-Marchesani syndrome is in many ways the opposite of Marfan's syndrome. This autosomal dominant disorder is characterized by short and fat extremities and dislocated lenses. The lenses are maldeveloped and spheroid, and they produce a lenticular myopia. Many of these patients are reported to develop progressive cardiovascular disease.

DISLOCATED LENS

The lens of the eye may become dislocated in many of the syndromes just described. Therefore a special description of this phenomenon is warranted.

The lens may be partially dislocated, or subluxed, when the zonular fibrils are weakened, stretched, or partially ruptured. The lens may be dislocated in any direction, as determined by where the residual fibrils are attached. As long as some of the fibrils remain attached to the lens, some part of the lens will remain behind the iris. Additional findings that occur with this problem are fluctuating astigmatism, iridodonesis, and monocular double vision. The latter is produced because some of the light rays are refracted through the lens while others pass around the edge of the lens.

If the zonule is completely broken, the lens can be completely dislocated. A lens floating freely in the vitreous can traumatize the retina, but more often the greatest problem is associated with degeneration of the lens material producing chronic intravitreal inflammation. An unattached lens can fall into the pupillary space; the lens is larger than the pupil and can completely occlude the opening, resulting in acute glaucoma. If the lens passes through the pupil into the anterior chamber, mechanical damage to the corneal endothelium and anterior chamber angle can occur.

REFERENCES

1. Duke-Elder WS: *System of Ophthalmology,* vol 3. St Louis, CV Mosby, 1967, p 333
2. Witkop CJ, Nance WE, Rawls RS, White JG: Autosomal recessive oculocutaneous albinism in man. Am J. Hum Genet 22:55, 1970
3. Lyon MD: Gene action in the X chromosome. Nature 190:372, 1961
4. Feman SS, Apt L, Roth AR: Nevus basal cell carcinoma syndrome. Am J Ophthalmol 78:222, 1974
5. Punnett HH, Harley RD: Genetics in Pediatric Ophthalmology, in Harley RD (ed): *Pediatric Ophthalmology.* WB Saunders, Philadelphia, 1975
6. McKusick VA: Heritable Disorders of Connective Tissue, vol 4. St Louis, CV Mosby, 1972
7. Fraumeni JF, Glass AG: Wilms' tumor and congenital aniridia. JAMA 206:825, 1968

Richard S. Smith, M. D.

3
External Disease

Congenital abnormalities and inflammatory disease are important concerns in any discussion of external ocular disease in children. In addition to these items, degenerations, dystrophies, pigmentations, and ocular manifestations of systemic disease in the conjunctiva, cornea, and iris will be reviewed here. Abnormalities of the lids and lacrimal system will be covered in Chapter 4.

CONGENITAL ABNORMALITIES

Conjunctiva

Primary tumors of the conjunctiva and cornea, such as melanomas and carcinomas, are rare in children. On the other hand, a number of tumorlike lesions occur on the conjunctiva, cornea, and iris as congenital findings. These may be composed of tissue elements found under normal conditions in a given location (hamartomas), or they may involve proliferation of cellular elements not normally found in the tissue (choristomas). Although such lesions may reach large size, as in neurofibromatosis, they are not neoplasms in the ordinary sense of the word. A number of syndromes characterized by multiple hamartomas were grouped by van der Hoeve into a loosely defined group known as the phakomatoses. This category includes neurofibromatosis, tuberous sclerosis, von Hippel-Lindau syndrome, and Sturge-Weber syndrome. Since most of the phakomatoses also have significant orbital manifestations, they will be discussed in a later chapter.

Papillomas are common lesions of the conjunctiva that involve the lids (tarsal conjunctiva) or globe (bulbar conjunctiva) in young individuals. Many papillomas are viral in origin, as is suggested by their tendency for contact spread. For example, a papilloma of the upper lid margin gives rise to a second papilloma in the corresponding contact area of the lower lid. Conjunctival papillomas may cause alarm because of their rate of growth and the frequent diffuse conjunctival involvement. The viral variety is prone to recur rapidly even after complete surgical excision, but this characteristic does not suggest malignancy. In a typical papilloma the conjunctival epithelium is thickened and shows multiple folds lined by fibrovascular connective tissue.[1,2]

Primary lymphangiomas and hemangiomas of the conjunctiva are uncommon hamartomatous lesions. Both capillary and cavernous hemangiomas are seen. Hemangiomatous tumors of the conjunctiva may also accompany the facial angiomas that are characteristic of Sturge-Weber syndrome or Rendu-Osler-Weber disease. This latter disorder is quite common, but the ocular findings are eclipsed by the problems associated with multiple angiomas of the gastrointestinal tract. Malignant vascular tumors of the conjunctiva are rare in children, although Kaposi's sarcoma has been reported.[1-3]

The most common choristomas involving the conjunctiva are dermoids and dermolipomas. Dermoids are solid white or yellow lesions typically located at the limbus, and they may involve the cornea. The histopathologic findings are variable and include dense connective tissue covered by epidermis. Hair follicles, sebaceous glands, and other skin appendages are often found within the substance of these benign tumors. Dermolipomas are frequently situated temporally and have a yellow appearance due to large amounts of fat. These tumors have no malignant growth potential and may produce a cosmetic problem or irregular astigmatism. Superficial keratectomy is usually a satisfactory means of surgical removal. Care should be taken, since deeper portions of the cornea or limbal area may be involved. Goldenhar's syndrome is an unusual congenital anomaly characterized by bilateral epibulbar dermoids, accessory auricular appendages, and aural fistulae. Many varieties of spinal abnormalities are seen in two-thirds of these patients. Lid and facial anomalies have been described.[1-3]

Episcleral osseous choristomas are uncommon lesions usually located in the superior temporal quadrant. They resemble conjunctival dermoids but they lack skin appendages or fat. The primary pathologic findings are deposits of dense normal bone.

Although lacrimal gland tissue is found normally in the orbit, ectopic lacrimal gland should be considered a choristoma when it occurs in places other than the lacrimal fossa. The orbit, conjunctiva, and lower lid may be sites of tumorlike deposits of normal lacrimal gland tissue.

Epithelial inclusion cysts of the conjunctiva are common, but they have little clinical significance. They may be found on either bulbar or tarsal conjunctiva, and they rarely grow to large size. Multiple cystic lesions are common. They may occur spontaneously or as sequelae to surgical closure of a conjunctival wound.[1-3]

Nevi of the conjunctiva often are apparent at birth, or they may become manifest during childhood. Thirty-five percent are evident clinically by the age of 9 years and 70 percent by the age of 30 years.[3] One-third of conjunctival nevi are unpigmented, and this may cause confusion with other conjunctival lesions. Nevi are most often found on the bulbar conjunctiva and the caruncle. All of the histologic varieties are seen in the conjunctiva, including junctional, compound, and dermal. There are two situations that may suggest growth. At puberty, a previously nonpigmented nevus can develop pigment, thus bringing the lesion to the attention of the patient for the first time. Epithelial inclusion cysts within a nevus also can enlarge, thus suggesting active growth. Conjunctival nevi are extremely common, but primary malignant melanoma of the conjunctiva is quite rare in children. Despite this fact, it should be remembered that approximately 40 percent of cases of malignant melanoma of the conjunctiva arise from preexisting conjunctival nevi. As with cutaneous melanomas, junctional or compound nevi are more likely to be precursors of malignant tumor than is a dermal nevus. The other type of congenital conjunctival pigmentation of importance in pediatrics is congenital conjunctival melanosis. This will be discussed in a later chapter along with other types of conjunctival and corneal pigmentations.[1,2,4]

Cornea

The most common congenital abnormality involving the size or shape of the cornea is microphthalmia, in which both the cornea and the rest of the ocular structures are much smaller than normal. Isolated microcornea, in which the corneal diameter is less than 11 mm but the remainder of the eye is normal in structure and dimensions, is less common. The curvature of such corneas often is increased greatly over the normal, thus producing marked myopia. This is in contrast to the situation with microphthalmia, where severe hypermetropia is the rule. Other ocular abnormalities demonstrated in eyes with microcornea include uveal colobomas and congenital cataracts. Scleralization of the cornea is seen in some individuals with microcornea, or it may appear as an independent finding; numerous family trees have been reported in the literature, and in most instances the defect has had an autosomal dominant inheritance pattern.[3]

The opposite situation from microcornea is megalocornea. There have been over 100 reports of this condition. The cornea is usually clear, but its diameter is greater than 13 mm. High degrees of astigmatism are common. Because of enlargement of the anterior segment, the iris may be stretched and atrophic. These alterations in the anterior segment may produce stretching of the zonules and luxation of the lens. If the lens becomes luxated, cataract or secondary glaucoma can occur. The condition is usually bilateral. Family trees have shown all varieties of dominant, recessive, and sex-linked inheritance. Megalocornea should not be confused with the buphthalmos of congenital glaucoma, which will be discussed in another chapter.[3]

In rare instances, corneal curvature is less than normal, a condition known as cornea plana. This may represent a variation of microcornea. The anterior chamber is shallow. This abnormality is associated with uveal colobomas, congenital cataract, retinal aplasia, and secondary glaucoma. Both dominant inheritance and recessive inheritance have been reported.[3]

Congenital hereditary corneal dystrophy is an uncommon condition that can also be confused with congenital glaucoma. There is diffuse opacity involving the full corneal thickness that is present at birth or shortly thereafter. The opacity is often sufficient to obscure all details of iris structure. Although progression is not a prominent feature, the opacity does increase with age. This condition also has a superficial resemblance to the mucopolysaccharidoses, but histologic study shows no abnormal deposits. The light microscopic and electron microscopic findings in this syndrome include minimal epithelial edema, disorganization of the stromal lamellae and a marked increase in diameter of stromal collagen fibrils, diffuse thickening of Descemet's membrane, and alterations of the organelles of the endothelium suggestive of defective function. There is a recessive inheritance pattern.[5]

A diverse group of uncommon congenital corneal opacities has been referred to as mesodermal dysgenesis of the iris and cornea, as well as anterior chamber cleavage syndrome, and they have been assigned a large and confusing number of eponyms. The pathogenesis and relationships among these different abnormalities are matters of considerable debate. The stepladder classification proposed by Waring et al.[6] is appealing in that it is based purely on anatomic findings. The name anterior chamber cleavage syndrome is perhaps preferable because it is easy to remember and it calls to mind the fact that different anomalies have common anatomic findings.

In terms of embryonic development of the anterior segment, there is not a true cleavage that results in formation of the anterior chamber. There are movements of primitive mesoderm and of the developing lens that may be faulty and may produce incomplete differentiation of anterior chamber structures. Three potential pathogenetic mechanisms have been proposed: (1) incomplete central migration of the mesoderm destined for corneal formation; (2) improper separation of the developing lens vesicle; (3) secondary anterior displacement of the lens-iris diaphragm.[6]

An additional point in support of a relationship among these diverse syndromes is that different variations of the cleavage syndrome may appear in the same family. For example, we observed a family in which the mother showed classic Axenfeld's anomaly without glaucoma. Her two male children were born with severe Peter's anomaly that included adhesion of the cataractous lens to the central corneal leukoma. Such families certainly suggest a common denominator in this group of diseases.

Waring et al.[6] divided the various syndromes into peripheral, central, and combined forms (Table 3-1). The most simple peripheral abnormality is posterior embryotoxon, in which there is a prominent Schwalbe's line, often visible on flashlight examination. This may be an isolated developmental anomaly not associated with congenital glaucoma. All of the other subdivisions of the cleavage syndrome often show concomitant congenital glaucoma, which will be discussed in greater detail in another chapter. If the prominent Schwalbe's line has iris processes attached to it, the name Axenfeld's anomaly is appropriate. About 50% of such patients develop juvenile glaucoma. Hypoplastic anterior iris stroma in combination with the two preceding anomalies is seen in the syndrome know as Rieger's anomaly. This malformation shows autosomal dominant inheritance with strong penetrance but marked variation in expression of the genetic defect. Abnormal shapes of the pupil are common, and there is persistence of the pupillary membrane. About 60 percent of these patients develop juvenile glaucoma. In some cases facial and dental abnormalities are seen.

The central abnormalities are more difficult to classify because of the dense corneal opacity that prevents visualization of anterior chamber structures. The mildest change is referred to as posterior keratoconus, although

Table 3-1
Anterior Chamber Cleavage Syndrome*

	Posterior Embryotoxon	Axenfeld's Anomaly	Rieger's Anomaly	Posterior Keratoconus	Peter's Anomaly
Prominent Schwalbe's line	+	+	+		
Potential glaucoma		+	+		+
Hypoplastic iris			+		
Posterior corneal depression				+	
Posterior corneal defect & leukoma					+
Iris adhesions to leukoma					+
Lenticular adhesions to leukoma					+

*Adapted from Waring et al.[6]

there is no relationship to typical anterior keratoconus. There is variable stromal haze overlying an indentation of Descemet's membrane. Despite this indentation, Descemet's membrane is present throughout. There may be other peripheral cleavage syndrome findings. Glaucoma is unusual.

The name Peter's anomaly refers to a variable syndrome that in its mildest form shows a central leukoma with a posterior corneal defect characterized by absence of Descemet's membrane and the corneal endothelium. In severe cases there are iris adhesions to the margin of the leukoma, and in the most severe cases a clear or cataractous lens is apposed or adherent to the corneal defect. Congenital glaucoma is frequent if there is lens involvement. There may be secondary shallowing of the anterior chamber and secondary glaucoma. Systemic anomalies including mental retardation, congenital heart disease, and urogenital abnormalities are often seen in these patients.

Iris

Early in the development of the optic vesicle a furrow develops along its inferior aspect that is referred to as the fetal or choroidal fissure. This furrow closes later in embryonic development and becomes the channel through which the intraocular blood supply and optic nerve develop. Either partial or complete failure of closure of this fissure results in the development of colobomas of the iris as well as the rest of the uvea and retina. Relative to other congenital ocular anomalies, colobomas are rather common. The severity of the coloboma depends on the extent of faulty closure of the fetal fissure. Colobomas that occur by this mechanism are called typical colobomas; they occur in the 6 o'clock position. This is often an isolated anomaly, and it may show a familial pattern. A coloboma may be complete or only an indentation at the pupillary border. Iris colobomas occur in other quadrants of the iris, although the pathogenesis is not always clear. The most commonly accepted theory is that atypical colobomas are caused by persistence of portions of the vascular pupillary membrane.

Persistence of remnants of the pupillary membrane is a frequent congenital abnormality. In the early months of fetal development this membrane is normally present. By 6 months it begins to atrophy, and normally it disappears. Tiny fragments may run across the pupil from one portion of the iris to another, usually attached at the collarette. Most commonly these remnants are bound only to the iris, but in some instances the lens and cornea are also involved.

Iris processes are attachments of the peripheral iris to the peripheral cornea or to Schwalbe's line; they are not remnants of the vascular pupillary membrane. They may occur as isolated findings or in association with congenital glaucoma or as one manifestation of the anterior chamber cleavage syndrome.

The name aniridia implies complete absence of the iris, but this degree of defect is actually a very uncommon abnormality. Most frequently the name is used to refer to marked iris hypoplasia in which there is a tiny stump of iris visible only on gonioscopy. The condition is usually bilateral, and photophobia is a universal symptom. Congenital nystagmus and poor visual acuity often accompany aniridia. Congenital cataracts, foveal hypoplasia, and juvenile glaucoma also occur. There is usually an autosomal dominant hereditary pattern, although recessive transmission occurs. Perhaps the most important point is that individuals with aniridia show a much higher incidence of Wilms' tumor than occurs in the general population (Miller's syndrome). Congenital renal abnormalities such as horseshoe kidney are also seen with aniridia. Because of the associated renal problems, any patient with aniridia should have an intravenous pyelogram to rule out these possibilities.[1,2]

Congenital iris nevi are as universal as cutaneous nevi. They account in considerable part for the variation in iris appearance between individuals. Iris nevi are more common in patients with neurofibromatosis, but this has no particular clinical significance. Nevi are usually located within the iris, although in rare instances they may be slightly elevated above the surface of the iris. The potential, especially in children, for transformation into malignant melanoma is extremely small. A nevus that shows a documented increase in size or produces abnormalities in the shape of the pupil is reason for suspicion of malignant transformation.

INFLAMMATORY DISEASE

Inflammatory disease involving the cornea, conjunctiva, and iris is common in the pediatric age group. This is a complex problem in terms of both diagnosis and classification. The clinical features and point of therapeutic attack vary considerably, depending on the etiologic agent. Before discussing the clinical features that characterize these diseases, the appropriate principles of therapeutics, and the specific causes of conjunctivitis and keratitis, it will be useful to review some general concepts.

Conjunctivitis and keratitis are associated with a wide variety of infectious agents, including bacteria, viruses, fungi, and parasites. Allergies, as well as physical and chemical stimuli, are the principal causes of noninfectious inflammation. The problem of inflammation involving the iris and the allied problems of chorioretinitis will be discussed in a later chapter.

When the physician is confronted with a patient with signs of conjuctival or corneal inflammation, a systematic evaluation is important. The patient may present with a wide variety of symptoms, including tearing, discharge, photophobia, foreign body sensation, pain, and visual disturbance. Absence of significant discharge suggests either allergy or viral infection. Decreased vision implies a greater or lesser degree of corneal involvement. Pain and photophobia may result from partial loss of corneal epithelium or from moderately severe keratitis and secondary iritis. The clinical history, including information about other infected family members or previous occurrences of similar bouts of inflammation, will be helpful in the differential diagnosis.

Careful examination of the affected eyes is also important. The first step is to determine if the inflammatory response is limited to the conjunctiva or to the cornea or if both structures are involved by the process. If only the corneal epithelium or Bowman's membrane is affected, the situation is usually of lesser concern than if deep corneal stroma is involved. A cellular response in the anterior chamber is a further indication of severe corneal disease. In some instances the conjunctival reaction may be limited to either the bulbar or tarsal conjunctiva or even to a localized area of the conjunctiva. The presence of papillae or follicles (*vide infra*) may give some indication of the nature of the inflammatory stimulus. Examination of the marginal tear strip with the slit lamp is helpful. In bacterial infections the severity of the inflammatory response usually produces a tear strip loaded with cells. In allergic or viral infections the cells suspended in the tears may be few, or there may be none.

Examination of a smear of conjunctival exudate and of scrapings taken from the cornea or conjunctiva is an important part of the diagnostic workup. The physician should acquire the habit of using appropriate staining procedures (Gram and Wright or Giemsa stains) (Table 3-2). Examination of the scraping often will yield important differential diagnostic information, and in the case of bacterial infections, knowledge of the presence of bacteria and their Gram-stain morphology may be vital for prompt institution of appropriate therapeutic measures. Wright or Giemsa stain may give additional indication of the etiology of the inflammation. Although cellular morphology should not be taken as an absolute indication of the involved agent, bacterial infections generally show high percentages of polymorphonuclear leukocytes, whereas viral infections have greater numbers of lymphocytes and mononuclear cells. Some viral infections are characterized by specific cytoplasmic or nuclear inclusions, although their demonstration and identification often require sophisticated knowledge and experience. Allergic reactions frequently show increased numbers of eosinophils and basophils in the smear.

Although initial therapy is usually instituted in bacterial infections after examination of the Gram-stained smear, appropriate cultures are important. In most institutions the hospital bacteriology laboratory is not always helpful, since they are not accustomed to dealing with the small samples of organisms provided by corneal and conjunctival scrapings, nor do they routinely encounter some of the infectious agents common in ophthalmology. Under the best of circumstances the culture media should be brought to the patient, and scrapings and swabs should be streaked out immediately on culture plates or

Table 3–2
Staining Techniques

Gram stain
1. Heat–fix smear
2. Flood slide with crystal violet; stain 1 min; wash with tap water
3. Flood slide with Gram's iodine; stain 1 min; wash with tap water
4. Decolorize 10–15 sec with 95% alcohol; wash with tap water
5. Counterstain with safranin

Wright stain (rapid, easy, readily available)
1. Unfixed slide—twelve drops Wright's blood stain
2. After 1 min, add 12 drops water
3. After 1 min, wash in tap water and dry

Giemsa stain (slower, better morphology)
1. Flood unfixed slide in methyl alcohol for 30 sec; drain and dry
2. Dilute 1 cc commercial Giemsa stock solution with 50 cc water; pH should be 6.8; stain for 45 min
3. Rinse with pH 6.8 buffer and dry

inoculated into liquid medium. If a fungal infection is suspected, specific culture media should be used (e.g., Sabouraud's medium). In this latter instance, a word of caution is indicated, since many hospital laboratory media contain inhibitors designed to prevent the growth of saprophytic fungal organisms. Many of these so-called nonpathogenic organisms produce severe keratitis, and their successful isolation requires the preparation of media without inhibitors. When obtaining material for cultures, the best samples are obtained by scraping the bed of a corneal ulcer or by scraping the conjunctiva with a platinum spatula. Sterile cotton swabs yield much lower percentages of positive cultures. In summary, the requirements for obtaining adequate cultures include direct supervision by the physician taking the culture, careful selection of appropriate media and properly harvested scrapings.[7]

Unless specially equipped laboratories are available, viral cultures are rarely useful. A strong prior suspicion of the specific virus is necessary to enable the virologist to work effectively in isolating it. In addition, acute and chronic serum samples are required for additional confirmation of a viral diagnosis.

Conjunctival and corneal inflammations show characteristics similar to those of inflammation elsewhere in the body, modified by the particular anatomic conditions that prevail in the anterior segment. With an acute inflammatory stimulus, conjunctival hyperemia appears. This represents a nonspecific vascular response to the inflammatory stimulus. Conjunctival hyperemia should not be confused with the dilation of the ciliary vessels (ciliary flush) seen in uveitis. The deep episcleral vessels that produce the ciliary flush will not show movement when the anesthetized conjunctiva is manipulated with a sterile swab. Dilated conjunctival vessels move freely with this technique. As is true elsewhere in the body, vasodilation is followed by leakage of fluid and cells. The conjunctiva is no exception, although the cornea behaves in a slightly different manner because of its compact construction. In the conjunctiva, fluid exudation from the dilated vessels produces chemosis (swelling). The type of cellular exudation depends on the inflammatory stimulus. The conjunctival stroma is infiltrated by inflammatory cells, and they also penetrate the conjunctival epithelium and produce an obvious external discarge that may accumulate at the inner canthus or may coat the lids and lashes. The clouding seen when the focus of inflammation is predominantly corneal is a combination of edema and infiltration by inflammatory cells. If the corneal inflammation is of sufficient severity, proteolytic enzymes released by leukocytes can excite a chemotactic reaction in the anterior chamber. This may produce an accumulation of cells in the inferior portion of the anterior chamber, a hypopyon. The presence of a hypopyon does not necessarily imply endophthalmitis or invasion of the eye by an infectious agent.

After the process of acute inflammation passes, or even during its evolution, a number of chronic changes may develop in the conjunctiva. Lymphoid follicles appear beneath the conjunctival epithelium in acute and chronic inflammation, producing a grayish velvety appearance. These structures are avascular, and on slit-lamp examination they are seen to be surrounded by small conjunctival vessels. Follicles typically occur on the tarsal conjunctiva, although the bulbar conjunctiva can also be involved.

Conjunctival papillae are seen in chronic inflammation. On slit-lamp examination they appear as elevated hyperplastic conjunctival epithelium with prominent central capillaries. Microscopic examination shows epithelial thickening and vascular dilation accompanied by a moderately severe inflammatory infiltrate.

With a severe inflammatory stimulus, membrane formation on the conjunctival surface may occur. A pseudomembrane consists of a network of fibrin and inflammatory cells that is easily separated from the epithelial surface. A true membrane is characterized by involvement of the epithelium by a similar type of exudation. Removal of a true membrane tears the conjunctival epithelium and produces bleeding.

If the inflammatory stimulus is localized (e.g., a foreign body), hypertrophic granulation tissue may appear on the bulbar or tarsal conjunctiva at the site of irritation. The bright reddish appearance and rapid growth may suggest a neoplasm. Pathologic examination shows dilated capillaries embedded in chronic inflammatory tissue, referred to as a pyogenic granuloma.

A final clinical manifestation of some types of conjunctivitis is the development of preauricular adenopathy. Although much has been written in the literature about Parinaud's oculoglandular syndrome, the name is applied so loosely that it has lost most of its original meaning. It should refer to ulcerative granulomatous conjunctivitis associated with preauricular adenopathy. One of the classic causes of such a reaction is cat-scratch fever.[3]

Although it is not the purpose of this chapter to discuss in detail the therapeutic management of inflammatory disease of the cornea and conjunctiva, it may be useful to make some general statements. The treatment of keratitis and conjunctivitis by many physicians tends to be too casual. Although it is true that conjuctivitis often improves in spite of treatment, in some cases inappropriate therapy may turn a simple situation into one that threatens vision. This problem warrants repetition of an old aphorism: Be sure of your diagnosis before you treat. Many drug companies are enthusiastic promoters of antibiotic and steroid combinations, and such dual medications frequently are provided in sample form. There are few types of ocular inflammation in which antibiotics and steroids are indicated at the same time, and when such a combination is used, very careful monitoring of the patient is mandatory.

Topical medications of whatever variety should be given in therapeutic dosage, not homeopathic dosage. In the case of ophthalmic drops, a single drop of medication is effectively eliminated from the conjunctival sac within about 20 min. If medication is given only three times per day, a therapeutic dose is present for only 1 hr out of 24 hr. If a bacterial infection is treated with antibiotics, minimal therapy requires that drops be given every 2 hr, with ointment applied at night. With a vision-threatening corneal ulcer, it may be necessary to increase the frequency to every 30 min, with hourly medication at night. Hospitalization is often necessary to ensure adequate treatment.

As with viral infections elsewhere in the body, viral conjunctivitis does not respond to antibiotics; thus they are contraindicated. Use of antibiotics in such circumstances may disturb the normal conjunctival flora and promote a secondary infection with resistant bacteria. The foreign-body sensation associated with viral keratoconjunctivitis is best relieved by use of a topical vasoconstrictor. This improves the appearance of the eyes, increases comfort, and allows the physician to avoid the pressure for nonindicated antibiotic therapy. With severe keratitis, a secondary anterior uveitis is often present. In such cases, topical mydriatics are helpful for relief of pain and photophobia. Finally, the physician should be concerned not only with personal hygiene but also with the sterility of diagnostic instruments after working with a patient with keratoconjunctivitis. Particularly in cases of viral infections, keratoconjunctivitis is often quite contagious. Epidemics often begin in the physician's office.

Bacterial Conjunctivitis and Keratitis

Bacterial conjunctivitis is not a common disease in children. The most frequently observed Gram-positive organisms are *Staphylococcus, Streptococcus,* and *Pneumococcus.* Gram-negative organisms that normally inhabit the intestinal tract may involve the eyes, although this is also quite unusual in children. *Haemophilus aegyptius* (Koch-Weeks bacillus) and *Moraxella lacunata* are two Gram-negative organisms that are particularly prone to involve the eye. Streptococcal and pneumococcal conjunctivitis in the acute form may produce a pseudomembrane. Some strains of pneumococcus can cause hemorrhagic conjunctivitis. Gonococcal conjunctivitis occurs in children but may produce only a mild purulent conjunctivitis. Spread in these cases is not usually by the venereal route. It should also be remembered that gonococcus is one of the few organisms capable of invading a normal cornea. Gonococcus is also one of the classic causes of ophthalmia neonatorum, a problem that will be discussed later in this chapter.

Generally, bacterial infections of the conjunctiva are easily treated, and as long as there is no corneal involvement, the sequelae are rarely serious. Bacterial corneal infections, in contrast, often produce devastating corneal changes with permanent visual loss. Because of this, the most careful diagnostic and therapeutic management is essential. *Staphylococcus* typically produces marginal corneal infiltrates or ulcerations. These primarily represent an allergic reaction to bacterial toxins. Such patients frequently have staphlococcal blepharitis. The blepharitis must be treated with antibiotics in order to eliminate the antigenic stimulus. The corneal infiltrates generally disappears promptly with short-term low-dosage therapy with corticosteroids. This is one of the rare instances where a combination of antibiotics and steroids is indicated.

A clinical point worth remembering is that only the gonococcus and diphtheria bacillus are capable of direct invasion through intact corneal epithelium. Therefore a bacterial cornea ulcer strongly suggests the possibility of preexisting corneal disease, systemic disease, or an incident of corneal trauma. If an apparently healthy patient develops a corneal ulcer in the absence of trauma, careful medical workup is indicated. As an example, the mild exposure of the cornea in the early stages of hyperthyroidism may damage the epithelium sufficiently that bacteria may invade the cornea and produce an ulcer.

Pneumococcal corneal ulcers frequently produce severe secondary iritis with hypopyon. They are rapidly progressive, and they often present as intracorneal abscesses; they may cause rapid melting of the cornea, with formation of a descemetocele and perforation. Vigorous antibiotic treatment is mandatory. Similar responses often are seen with *Pseudomonas* and *Proteus* infections.

Because the process of inflammation and repair associated with bacterial corneal ulcers is likely to produce permanent visual loss, all corneal ulcers must be treated as potential threats to vision. Due to the rapid growth of organisms such as *Pneumococcus* and *Pseudomonas,* treatment cannot await the results of cultures. This emphasizes the importance of proper preparation and staining of smears, as mentioned earlier in this chapter.

Bacterial corneal ulcers may be treated by three approaches: topical, subconjunctival, and intravenous medication. Initial antibiotic selection depends on the Gram stain. Many therapeutic regimens have been tried, and the suggestions proposed by Jones[7] (Table 3-3) are useful. If no organisms are found on the Gram stain, or if there are Gram-positive organisms, topical bacitracin and gentamicin are combined with systemic methicillin. For Gram-negative cocci, topical bacitracin drops and systemic penicillin are suggested. Gram-negative rods are treated topically, subconjunctivally, and systemically by a combination of gentamicin and carbenicillin. The therapeutic selection of these drugs for initial therapy is a conservative approach based on the worst possible case. All three routes of administration are not necessary in all cases. It is obvious that the results of culture and sensitivity tests or the patient's clinical course may demand an alteration in the initial drug selection. Repeated cultures after a period of therapy are essential to document sterilization of the ulcer. Closely supervised treatment with topical corticosteroids after a few days of antibiotic therapy helps decrease the inflammatory response and scar tissue formation. Except in unusual circumstances, it is often best to hospitalize a patient with a central corneal ulcer to assure a satisfactory treatment response and to make certain that corneal thinning and perforation do not ensue.

Contact Lenses

The wearing of contact lenses is increasingly common in teenagers, and with special indications, infants and children may be fitted with contact lenses. This problem is discussed here because the principal serious complication of wearing contact lens is infection. Although both hard lenses and soft lenses are worn by those in the pediatric age group, the latter are most often encountered. Despite warnings in the older literature and in some cases on the package insert accompanying soft contact lenses, there is little contraindication to use of topical eye medications. Prescription and proprietery preparations containing epinephrine derivatives should be avoided because many of these products have a tendency to produce permanent discoloration of soft

Table 3–3
Initial Antibiotic Selection*

Gram Stain	Topical	Systemic†
No identifiable organisms	Bacitracin/gentamicin	Methicillin/gentamicin
Gram-positive cocci or rods	Bacitracin/gentamicin	Methicillin
Gram-negative cocci	Bacitracin	Penicillin G
Gram-negative rods	Gentamicin/carbenicillin	Gentamicin/carbenicillin

*Adapted from Jones.[7]

†Intravenous and subconjunctival therapy is used only with careful ophthalmic supervision for severe ulcers.

contact lenses. If it is necessary to use topical fluorescein stain to demonstrate corneal pathology, the soft contact lens should first be removed; the staining procedure should be followed by copious irrigation of the conjunctival sac to prevent staining of the contact lens with fluorescein. Other topical medications may be used with impunity, and there is no firm clinical evidence that medications are concentrated to toxic levels within soft contact lenses. The possibility of corneal abrasion with soft or hard contact lenses is one of the risks of wearing these devices. As mentioned previously, corneal abrasion often provides a route of invasion for infectious organisms. For this reason the fitting and wearing of contact lens should be carefully supervised by an ophthalmologist. Any suspicion of injury is reason for referral and careful evaluation of the possibility of infectious disease.

Viral Infections

The TRIC viruses provide a logical point of transition between discussion of bacterial infections and discussion of viral infections, since they are large and rather atypical viruses that resemble bacteria in some respects, including their sensitivity to antibiotics. Although trachoma is rarely seen in this country, it still is one of the leading causes of blindness throughout the world. Trachoma is a chronic disease that begins in childhood and has the conjunctival epithelium and corneal epithelium as its primary targets. Marked follicular and papillary hyperplasia occurs. The corneal involvement becomes manifest as pannus (vascularization) that begins superiorly and extends with stromal scarring into the visual axis. Conjunctival involvement produces severe scarring of the lids, with entropion formation. This is a contagious disease intimately associated with poor personal hygiene. Corneal scrapings show intracytoplasmic inclusion bodies. Sulfonamides, tetracycline, and erythromycin applied topically are all effective against the virus. Reinfection, inadequate treatment, and poor follow-up make the disease difficult to eradicate in endemic areas.

The other TRIC virus of importance in the pediatric age group is that causing inclusion conjunctivitis. This agent produces a follicular conjunctivitis with a prolonged course. Scarring and pannus formation occur, although they are less common than in trachoma. Infection of both ocular and genital mucosa is seen. This virus is also a cause of ophthalmia neonatorum. The same antibiotics used for trachoma are effective. There is some argument that trachoma and inclusion conjunctivitis are caused by different strains of the same virus.

Herpes simplex virus occurs in two forms: HSV-II involves primarily a genital infection, whereas HSV-I involves the skin or eyes. Cutaneous involvement is far more common, but the ocular disease produces serious visual disturbance. Corneal herpes begins as a punctate epithelial keratitis. These lesions coalesce to form a typical dendritic figure that stains with fluorescein. At this stage the viral infection is usually highly susceptible to treatment with specific antiviral agents. The problem with herpes simplex is its tendency to produce recurrent attacks. These attacks may occur months or years after the primary infection. With each recurrent attack the danger of corneal stromal involvement increases. The stromal involvement usually produces permanent stromal scarring and visual loss. Stromal herpes is often accompanied by anterior uveitis. Corneal sensation is decreased.

The treatment of herpes simplex keratitis varies depending on the stage and severity of the disease. In most cases idoxuridine (5-iodo-2'-deoxyuridine, IDU) is used topically as drops or ointment; this usually results in healing of epithelial herpes in 5–7 days. IDU is a pyrimidine analog that causes the production of defective viral DNA. It may produce side effects, including punctate epithelial keratitis, occlusions of the lacrimal punctum, and conjunctival scarring. True allergies to the drug also occur. Some viral strains are resistent to IDU. If the ulcer does not heal within a reasonable time, two alternatives are available. The old treatment for epithelial keratitis was debridement (scraping) of the infected epithelium. Although this treatment is not as popular as it once was, it is still quite effective. Vidarabine, a new antiviral agent, has recently been released to the market and is available as 3 percent ophthalmic ointment. It has some theoretical advantages in that whereas IDU is metabolically inactivated, vidarabine metabolic products retain their antiviral activity. Both IDU and vidarabine are also useful in the treatment of stromal keratitis. Since there is strong evidence that stromal herpes is primarily an immunologic reaction to viral protein, the carefully controlled use of corticosteroids in combination with antivirals is indicated. There is some evidence in individuals with recurrent stromal keratitis that prophylactic treatment with low doses of steroids and antivirals is useful in reducing the incidence of recurrent attacks. Such treatment demands careful supervision. Despite treatment, corneal scarring may develop with visual loss. Penetrating keratoplasty often is needed to restore vision.

External involvement by varicella zoster virus is a rare occurrence in children. When it happens, severe stromal damage with permanent scarring and visual loss is a potential problem. In herpes zoster keratitis there is often severe anterior uveitis that produces multiple complications, including secondary glaucoma, anterior and posterior synechiae, and cataract.

Adenovirus infections of the conjunctiva and cornea are common in both children and adults. Numerous serological types of adenoviruses have been described. Pharyngoconjunctival fever is classically associated with adenovirus type 3, although a similar clinical picture is seen with other adenoviruses. This disease is characterized by fever, pharyngitis, and follicular conjunctivitis associated with swollen lymph nodes. It is highly infectious and may persist for several days. Nonspecific treatment with vasoconstrictor agents is the only therapeutic possibility.

Epidemic keratoconjunctivitis (EKC) was originally associated with adenovirus type 8, but other adenoviruses produce similar clinical findings. Both children and adults are affected by this disease, which presents two different clinical pictures. In some parts of the United States, EKC has an acute onset with marked conjunctival injection, chemosis, and preauricular adenopathy. There may be moderate discharge with pseudomembrane formation. At this stage the cornea is clear, and corneal infiltrates do not appear until 1–2 weeks after the onset of inflammation. The conjunctival inflammation typically disappears within a few weeks, but the corneal lesions persist for some time thereafter. Mydriatics and patching are suggested as the only treatment. In the other form of EKC the onset may be less acute, with less prominent conjunctival reaction. Such patients present with decreased vision, photophobia, severe foreign-body sensation, and numerous small subepithelial lesions at the level of Bowman's membrane. The margins of the lesions are fuzzy and poorly defined. The visual disability as well as the symptoms in this second form of EKC may be extremely disabling. In such cases topical corticosteroids are the initial treatment of choice. The infection can persist for many months, and there is a strong tendency for recurrent attacks if steroid therapy is tapered. Some ophthalmologists have suggested that steroids should not be used, and this may well be true with the acute presentation. When there is severe visual loss and disabling photophobia, it does not seem to be in the best interest of the patient to withhold steroid therapy. Antiviral agents are not effective in adenovirus infections.[3]

On rare occasions accidental infections of the eye with vaccinia virus occur following vaccination, producing severe keratitis with permanent corneal scarring. IDU, interferon, and topical immune serum have all been suggested as treatments for this unusual complication.

Verrucae and molluscum contagiosum lesions on the lids may cause secondary keratoconjunctivitis. In both cases the chronic irritation is produced by keratin debris and viral particles falling into the conjunctival sac. The only effective treatment is surgical removal of the lid lesion.

Fungal Infections

Keratomycosis is a potentially serious cause of visual loss, but it occurs primarily in adults and only rarely in children. In most instances fungal infections of the cornea are seen in situations in which there is a history of injury or in eyes damaged by previous inflammation. There is certainly a possibility of corneal trauma in children, but in actual clinical practice few cases of keratomycosis are seen. Careful corneal scrapings and appropriate fungal stains are needed to make the diagnosis. A child may require general anesthesia to obtain adequate material for scrapings and culture, since the fungi are often absent from the superficial cornea. Conjunctival infection with *Candida* species can occur in children, but it is uncommon. Nystatin (500,000 units/cc) is useful for *Candida,* but it has no therapeutic potential for other fungal organisms. At this time the only other readily available topical antifungal agent is amphotericin B, which may be used topically as 0.5 percent solution. Natamycin (Pimaricin) is available from the manufacturer on special request.

Allergy

Allergic reactions of the conjunctiva and cornea take several forms. Most common are diffuse conjunctival hyperemia, itching, and tearing that often are related to pollen or other allergens suspended in the air. Usually the only corneal reaction is a punctate epithelial keratitis. In most cases elimination of the allergen is impractical, and treatment relies on medications that produce symptomatic relief, including vasoconstrictors, systemic antihistamines, and topical steroids. Because of their potential side effects on intraocular pressure and increased susceptibilty to infectious disease, steroids should be used only in severe cases, and then with careful supervision.

Atopic eczema can produce a variety of complications in the rare instances of ocular involvement. The most common manifestation is punctate epithelial keratitis related to keratin scales falling into the conjunctival sac from the affected lids. Increased incidences of cataract and keratoconus are also seen in patients with atopic eczema. The development of keratoconus may be related to local trauma due to repeated rubbing of the lids.

Prolonged exposure to a variety of chemicals including ophthalmic drugs can produce a contact allergy involving the lids and conjunctiva. Atropine, pilocarpine, and topical anesthetics are most often involved. The sensitivity may be related to preservatives or vehicles in which a drug is dissolved rather than to the drug itself. In cases where continued treatment is necessary, a preparation from a different manufacturer may relieve the problem.

Theodore developed the concept of microbiallergic conjunctivitis, and the most common manifestation of this condition is staphylococcal marginal corneal infiltrates. The acute sensitivity of these infiltrates to corticosteroids is further evidence of their allergic nature. Phlyctenular keratitis is also most likely an allergic reaction to bacterial products. As is indicated by one of the old names referring to this condition, scrofulous ophthalmia, the primary pathogen for many years was considered to be tuberculosis. Phlyctenules have been produced experimentally with extracts of tuberculoprotein. This supports the hypothesis that this is a mechanism in humans even though mycobacteria have not been found in the lesions and the histopathology does not resemble that of a tubercle. By far the most common cause of phlyctenules is staphylococcal allergy, although they have been reported with other bacteria as well. The lesion begins near the limbus and may spread onto the cornea, bringing vascularization with it. The elevated phlyctenule can migrate over a period of time, producing corneal thinning and scarring in the visual axis. The reaction to corticosteroids is favorable, but there is a tendency for the lesions to recur. Specific treatment of any infection invloving the lids is indicated.[3]

A peculiar kind of inflammation that primarily affects the cornea is interstitial keratitis. The vast majority of cases of interstitial keratitis are secondary to congenital syphilis. There is diffuse corneal inflammation, somewhat concentrated in the deep stroma. In the initial stages there is often severe anterior uveitis. This is one of the late manifestations of hereditary syphilis; although it may occur in adults, it is most often seen in teenagers. Other stigmata of congenital syphilis are often present. This most likely represents an immune response to treponemal antigens, but organisms are not found in the cornea during the acute phases of inflammation. The end result is diffuse corneal scarring with vascularization and loss of vision. The inflammatory response eventually subsides, leaving an opacified cornea with ghost vessels. This may eventually require penetrating keratoplasty to restore vision. Since syphilitic interstitial keratitis may occur in patients who have negative VDRL findings, the FTAabs test must be done if syphilis is suspected. In addition, interstitial keratitis has also been ascribed to tuberculosis infections, mumps, and trypanosomiasis. Cogan described an unusual syndrome characterized by nonsyphilitic interstitial keratitis with vestibuloauditory symptoms. This usually occurs in young adults, but cases have been reported as early as 4.5 years of age.[3]

Ophthalmia neonatorum is discussed separately from other infections because it presents a problem of particular interest for pediatricians. In a general way the name refers to bilateral conjunctivitis seen in the perinatal period. Infection usually occurs during the process of birth. Many varieties of bacteria have been isolated in such cases, including staphylococci, pneumococci, and gonococci. Viral inclusion conjunctivitis (*Chlamydia*) accounts for anywhere from 10 percent to 30 percent of cases. As in other types of infectious disease involving the anterior segment, cultural confirmation of the diagnosis is essential for appropriate treatment. Prophylaxis with either silver nitrate or antibiotics at the time of birth is of questionable value, especially if treatment of limited duration is given. Any discharge from the eyes of a newborn child should immediately be cultured and Gram-stained, and the appropriate antibiotic should be chosen as described earlier in this chapter.

Vernal conjunctivitis was succinctly described by Duke-Elder[3] as "a recurrent bilateral inflammation of the conjunctiva, of periodic seasonal incidence . . . and unknown etiology." The tarsal conjunctiva is most commonly affected with large papillae that also may involve the limbal conjunctiva. Patients complain of redness, itching, tearing, and mucoid discharge. Smears of the discharge often show many eosinophils. Vernal conjunctivitis is usually a disease of late spirng and summer, and it rarely affects adults. Much has been written about the etiology of this disease, but little solid information exists. It is presumed to be an allergic manifestation because of its seasonal incidence and its response to steroids. Important corneal changes are uncommon, but superficial vascularization occurs. The incidence of this disease varies considerably in different parts of the country. Intensive corticosterioid therapy is helpful, but the side effects of these topical agents create problems. Despite the difficulty of doing so in children, it is important to monitor the intraocular pressure to make sure that the patient is not a steroid responder.

Trauma

The potential effects of blunt or penetrating trauma to the anterior segment of the globe mandate that all such patients be seen promptly by an ophthalmologist. Even relatively minor blunt ocular trauma may produce hyphema, and the complications of such bleeding have grave prognostic significance. The blunt trauma that causes this bleeding may produce a tear of the iris and damage to the anterior chamber angle stuctures. This, in turn, may cause acute traumatic glaucoma, as well as a late-onset type of glaucoma that will be discussed in greater detail in another chapter. The vascular damage that produces the bleeding may set up a situation in which rebleeding may occur after a few days. Massive rebleeding may also result in elevated intraocular pressure and the possibility of corneal blood staining (see section on pigmentation). For all of these reasons, hospitalization is often recommended to ensure that the patient has complete bed rest with sedation and binocular patching. It is believed that these measures reduce the incidence of rebleeding. The use of mydriatics or miotics does not appear to be of clinical benefit.

A common type of corneal trauma that the pediatrician may have to treat is a corneal abrasion. In the majority of cases, 24 hr of patching with antibiotic ointment are sufficient to heal the abrasion without complication. However, it should be borne in mind that any abrasion is a potential portal of entry for infectious agents and should not be treated in a casual fashion. Trauma with vegetable matter carries a particular risk of bacterial or fungal infection; such patients should be followed carefully. Corneal abrasions produced by a comb or fingernail often cause disproportionate inflammatory reactions with severe keratitis and iritis that require the application of mydriatics, antibiotics, and in some instances steroids. Steroids should be used only with careful follow-up because of the risk of potentiating a secondary infection. Ultraviolet burns of the cornea are rarely seen in the younger pediatric age group, but preteens and teenagers often develop them after careless use of sunlamps. These cause diffuse keratitis with marked corneal epithelial damage and have the same symptoms as a severe corneal abrasion. Bilateral patching with mydriatics often is necessary. Usually these lesions heal within 24–48 hr with no permanent damage.

Chemical burns of the cornea and conjunctiva are more commonly seen in adults, but because of their devastating effects on vision and the great importance of prompt first-aid measures, they must be emphasized here. Many common household products including drain and oven cleaners, bleaches, and numerous cosmetic agents, are either strongly alkaline or acidic due to any of a wide range of active ingredients. Governmental regulation has been less than ideal in terms of package warnings and elimination of unneecessarily toxic products from the consumer market. For an unknown product, the best source of information is usually a poisin control center. Package labels, especially those for cosmetics, cannot be depended on for chemical content or for the degree of potential danger on occular exposure. Acid and alkali burns differ considerably in their mechanisms of action and prognoses. Organic and inorganic acids cause instantaneous damage, with coagulation of superficial protein and negligible penetration into the eye. Alkaline substances, on the other hand, continue to produce damage as long as they are in contact with the eye; they readily penetrate the ocular coats, with not only corneal damage but also severe damage to the iris, lens, and anterior segment of the globe. In all cases of chemical injury to the eye, the treatment of choice is prompt irrigation. This is usually facilitated by adding a topical anesthetic. Prior to irrigation, a simple broad-range pH paper should be dipped into the conjunctival sac to ascertain the beginning pH. Once this is done, irrigation with large quantities of solution should begin and should continue until the pH has become neutral. The particular irrigating solution is not important, and specific efforts at neutralization of an acid or alkaline substance are not worthwhile. Sterile 5 percent sodium chloride solution is almost universally available in offices and emergency rooms and is as satisfactory as anything. Lacking even this, ordinary tap water is better than nothing. The conjunctival pH should be checked again 30 min after irrigation has been discontinued. Often there will be sufficient leaching of material from inside the eye to elevate the pH again. If this occurs, further irrigation is indicated. If the toxic agent is solid or semisolid, both lids should be carefully everted to make sure that particulate matter is not lodged beneath the lids, where considerable additional damage can take place. Once the emergency irrigation has been completed, all such patients should promptly be referred to an ophthalmologist; if this is not done, further sequelae of injury may include infection, corneal ulceration, stromal melting, perforation, and endophthalmitis. The details of treatment to avoid or deal with these complications are beyond the scope of this book.

DEGENERATIONS AND DYSTROPHIES

The terms *degeneration* and *dystrophy* are used extensively in ophthalmology to organize our thinking on a wide variety of diseases. When properly used, the term *degeneration* describes the tissue reaction to a disease process. In contrast, the term *dystrophy* usually refers to a bilateral tissue change with characteristic histopathologic features and often a strong family history. Many of the degenerations and dystrophies are of primary concern in adults and will not be covered in this section unless the early manifestations occur in children.

Xerosis refers to excessive drying of the conjunctiva and cornea, and this produces keratinization. Most newborn infants produce very few tears; it has been observed that only 35 percent have normal rates of secretion. This failure of tear secretion usually disappears within a few weeks, but it may persist, with severe drying of the conjunctiva and cornea. In some instances this alacrima may have a neurogenic basis and may be accompanied by other signs of brain damage. Other cases have been related to lacrimal gland aplasia. The Riley-Day syndrome has defective lacrimation as one of the primary signs of autonomic insufficiency. In these patients the defect is bilateral and may result in photophobia and corneal ulceration. Another cause of congenital alacrima is the syndrome known as anhidrotic ectodermal dysplasia. All of these possibilities are distinctly unusual.[8] On the other hand, xerophthalmia secondary to vitamin A deficiency is a worldwide public health problem of great magnitude. This may lead to corneal melting or keratomalacia, in association with other vitamin and protein deficiencies. The incidence is high in areas where nutrition is poor, and vitamin A deficiency is an important cause of blindness in many parts of the world. It may be induced in patients who limit themselves to bizarre organic diets.[9]

Band keratopathy is a calcific degeneration of Bowman's membrane that often follows intraocular disease such as uveitis, keratitis, or longstanding glaucoma. Although it is more common in adults than in children, it is often seen in individuals with childhood uveitis. The opacity appears as a horizontal band across the visual axis and is usually due to calcium deposits. It is often possible to remove the calcium chemically and surgically, with considerable improvement in visual acuity.

Primary degenerations of the iris are less common and are seen most frequently following trauma. The iris may become atrophic or distorted by scar tissue. Essential iris atrophy is a slowly progressive loss of iris tissue that eventually results in a severe, refractory, secondary glaucoma. Whereas such problems arise primarily in adults, cases have been noted as early as 5 years of age. Essential iris atrophy is often unilateral, but it may involve both eyes. A few family trees have been described, but generally the disease appears as an isolated problem.[10]

There are numerous corneal dystrophies that affect the adult population but are relatively infrequent in the pediatric age group. The least controversial classification of the dystrophies is geographic. The anterior membrane dystrophies (epithelium and Bowman's dystrophies) are for the most part quite rare, with one exception. Cogan's microcystic dystrophy (dystrophic recurrent erosion, map-dot-fingerprint dystrophy) is the most common form of anterior membrane corneal dystrophy seen in routine ophthalmic practice. It has a variable appearance that changes over a period of time. It is characterized by bilateral cystic or linear patterns limited to the corneal epithelium. At one time or another, approximately 30 percent of patients with this problem develop symptoms typical of recurrent corneal erosion, with pain, tearing, and photophobia. This is usually a sporadic disease, but it may be transmitted as an autosomal dominant. Because of the tendency for recurrent erosions, such patients should be followed carefully by an ophthalmologist.[11]

The classic corneal dystrophies, which include granular, lattice, and macular dystrophies, are all diseases that involve primarily the corneal stroma, with secondary changes in the epithelium (Table 3-4). Granular dystrophy has an autosomal dominant hereditary pattern, with typical lesions in the central cornea. Although these lesions may appear in children, visual symptoms are rare until later in life.

Macular dystrophy, on the other hand, has an autosomal recessive inheritance pattern; it shows multiple poorly defined grayish central opacities that often reduce visual acuity during the childhood and teenage years. In addition, due to secondary involvement of the epithelium, there is a tendency to develop a recurrent erosion syndrome with severe pain and disability; because of this and because of the effects on vision, corneal transplantation is often necessary early in adult life.

Lattice dystrophy is an autosomal dominant disease affecting the corneal stroma; it presents with linear opacities that eventually become diffuse, with an appearance resembling macular dystrophy. This disease also causes recurrent erosions, with an early decrease in vision that requires keratoplasty.

Other corneal dystrophies are rare during childhood. Although Fuchs' combined endothelial dystrophy is a common problem in older adults, it is rarely if ever seen in children. Visual disability is not a problem until later in life.

Posterior polymorphous dystrophy is characterized by irregular pits and opacities, with opacification in the deep layers of corneal stroma and Descemet's membrane. This condition shows both autosomal dominant and recessive inheritance, but despite its striking appearance on slit-lamp examination, it rarely causes visual disability.

Keratoconus produces an axial bulging of the cornea that eventually may cause high degrees of astigmatism, with vision correctable only by contact lenses. Young children rarely show typical changes, and the disease usually develops first during the teenage years. There is not a prominent hereditary pattern, and many cases are isolated. Although the disease is invariably bilateral, it may be extremely asymmetric during the early stages. With sufficient stretching of the cornea, tears in Descemet's membrane develop, with leakage of fluid into the cornea accompanied by iritis and pain. This condition is known as acute hydrops, and it usually resolves, leaving further opacity and stretching of the cornea. Ultimately, keratoplasty may be necessary, but the course of the disease is so variable in different individuals that it is difficult to give a specific prognosis. There is an increased incidence of keratoconus in atopic dermatitis, vernal conjunctivitis, and Down's syndrome.

SYSTEMIC DISEASE

The general features of the mucopolysaccharidoses (MPS) were discussed in Chapter 2. The list of diseases that properly fall in this group continues to grow each year. From the viewpoint of external disease, the common denominator of most of the mucopolysaccharidoses is diffuse corneal clouding, frequently present at birth. Although they are nonprogressive, there may be severe visual changes. Deposits of the abnormal mucopolysaccharide are found in the corneal epithelium, stroma, or endothelium. The Hunter and

Table 3–4
Staining Patters of Corneal Dystrophies

	Masson	Colloidal Iron	PAS	Amyloid	Birefringence
Granular	+	−	−	−	−
Macular	−	+	−	−	−
Lattice	+	−	+	+	+

Sanfilippo syndromes do not have corneal clouding, nor does MPS-VII. The clinical features, genetics, and enzymology of these diseases have been well summarized by Yanoff and Fine.[2]

Corneal clouding similar to that seen in the mucopolysaccharidoses is also seen in some of the mucolipidoses, in which retinal pathology is the dominant feature. Mucolipidoses type I and type III and Gm_1-gangliosidosis type I are most often associated with corneal clouding. These are all rare syndromes, as are the sphingolipidoses. These latter diseases have their principle effects on the retina, except for Fabry's disease, where whorl-like opacities are seen in the deeper layers of the corneal epithelium. In all of these diseases, electron microscopic examination reveals lipid-containing inclusions of various morphologic types.[2]

Cystinosis is usually inherited with an autosomal recessive pattern, and it appears in both infantile and adult forms. The adult form is an isolated corneal defect without significance to the patient. On the other hand, childhood cystinosis is associated with dwarfism and progressive renal dysfunction. As far as the eyes are concerned, deposits of cystine crystals can be seen with a slit lamp in the cornea, and they occur in many other parts of the eye. These deposits have no effect on visual acuity, but they are interesting clinical findings and may be helpful in the differential diagnosis of this disease.

Primary pemphigus and benign mucosal pemphigoid are rare diseases in adults and probably do not occur in children. The few cases described in children most likely are examples of erythema multiforme (Stevens-Johnson syndrome). In some cases the etiology is unknown, but often there is a connection with idiopathic drug reactions. When the eye is involved, changes similar in pathology to those occurring elsewhere in the body involve the conjunctival and corneal epithelium. Scarring of the lid and adhesions between the bulbar conjunctiva and tarsal conjunctiva are common complications. In addition, there usually is cessation of tear formation, with a severely dry eye.

The well-known triad of urethritis, conjunctivitis, and polyarthritis is referred to in the literature as Reiter's syndrome. The clinical triad explains most of the patient's symptoms. The iritis may be severe and can be treated in conventional fashion. This is primarily a disease of older patients, but cases have been reported in children.[12]

Xeroderma pigmentosum is a rare disease that begins in childhood and is characterized by extreme cutaneous sensitivity to light. Chronic exposure to sunlight results in the development of basal and squamous cell carcinomas, as well as malignant melanomas of the skin. The conjunctiva and lids are frequently involved.

A number of systemic diseases may affect the iris. Focal infiltrates and hemorrhages are seen in childhood leukemia. In the various glycogenoses, infiltration of the iris and iris pigment epithelium with the abnormal storage material may occur. Although it is rare, iris involvement in the histiocytoses has been reported. A syndrome perhaps related to the histiocytoses is juvenile xanthogranuloma, which is characterized by tissue infiltration with histiocytes and giant cells containing considerable amounts of lipid. The iris may be involved, with formation of new iris vessels and a tendency for spontaneous hyphema. Although this disease is unusual, it should be kept in mind in the differential diagnosis of a child with a spontaneous hyphema.

PIGMENTATION

Pigmentation of the cornea and conjunctiva may be caused by metallic compounds, drug deposits, and a variety of endogenous pigmented products. A retained intraocular metallic foreign body can produce deposits of iron or copper in the cornea or conjunctiva, depending on its location. Naturally occurring deposits of iron in the corneal epithelium are seen on slit-lamp examination as superficial focal or linear brownish deposits. In the pediatric age group the most common corneal iron line is a Fleischer ring, a circular deposit around the periphery of the deformed cornea in keratoconus. This should not be confused with a Kayser-Fleischer ring, which consists of endogenous copper deposits in patients with Wilson's disease. This latter usually is not seen until after several years of involvement with the disease, and it is unlikely in young children.

Various epinephrine products are used for the treatment of glaucoma, including congenital glaucoma. Long-term use of these drugs may produce local deposits of adrenochrome pigmentation on the cornea or in the conjunctiva. These should not be confused with malignant melanoma. Long-term high dosage with phenothiazine derivatives also produces a diffuse brownish pigmentation of cornea and conjunctiva.

Numerous endogenous pigmentations are also possible. In a patient who has suffered severe hyphema accompanied by elevated intraocular pressure, the hemosiderin from the degenerating blood in the anterior chamber may cause severe blood staining of the cornea, with a marked decrease in visual acuity. This is one of the principal reasons for careful ophthalmic follow-up of hyphema. The other significant conjunctival pigmentation, melanosis oculi, is actually a congenital lesion, although it may not become manifest in striking fashion until puberty. Congenital melanosis oculi may involve all parts of the eye. If the pigment is limited to the uveal tract and the conjunctiva, it is referred to as ocular melanosis. If the skin of the eye-lids and surrounding face is also involved, oculocutaneous melanosis is present, also known as the nevus of Ota. Although malignant transformation in all of these congenital melanin abnormalities has been reported, it is extremely rare and highly unlikely in children.[3]

Pigmentary abnormalities of the iris may be referred to generically as heterochromia. This designation takes in a considerable differential diagnosis. The term heterochromia refers to a difference in color between the two eyes and implies an increase in pigmentation or a decrease in pigmentation of the abnormal eye relative to the normal eye. In most instances the causes of heterochromia are individually rare, and congenital heterochromia may be isolated or associated with Wardenburg's syndrome or Romberg's syndrome. Acquired heterochromia is seen after trauma (hyphema/iris atrophy), with melanosis oculi, and with neoplastic or histiocytic involvement of the iris.[13]

REFERENCES

1. Hogan MJ, Zimmerman LE: Ophthalmic Pathology. Philadelphia, WB Saunders, 1962
2. Yanoff M, Fine BS: Ocular Pathology. New York, Harper & Row, 1975
3. Duke-Elder S: System of Ophthalmology, vol VIII, Diseases of the Outer Eye. London, Henry Kimpton, 1965
4. Reese AB Tumors of the Eye (ed 3). New York, Harper & Row, 1976
5. Kenyon KR, Maumenee AE: The histologic and ultrastructural pathology of congenital hereditary corneal dystrophy. Invest Ophthalmol 7:475, 1968
6. Waring GO, Rodriguez MM, Laibson PR: Anterior chamber cleavage syndrome. A stepladder classification. Surv Ophthalmol 20:3, 1975
7. Jones DB: Early diagnosis and therapy of bacterial corneal ulcers. Int Ophthalmol Clin 13:1–29, 1973
8. Smith RS, Maddox SF, Collins BE: Congenital alacrima. Arch Ophthalmol 79:45–48, 1968
9. Smith RS, Farrell T, and Bailey T: Keratomalacia. Surv Ophthalmol 20:213–219, 1975
10. Duke-Elder S: System of Ophthalmology, vol IX, Diseases of the Uveal Tract. London, Henry Kimpton, 1966
11. Rodriguez MM, Fine BS, Laibson PR, Zimmerman LE: Disorders of the corneal epithelium. Arch Ophthalmol 92:475, 1974
12. Vergnani RJ, Smith RS: Reiter syndrome in a child. Arch Ophthalmol 91:165–166, 1974
13. Gladston RM: Development and significance of heterochromia of the iris. Arch Neurol 21:184, 1969

Richard S. Smith, M.D.

4
Lids, Orbit, and Lacrimal System

CONGENITAL ANOMALIES

Malformations that involve the lid and orbit present a problem in classification because so many variations and combinations of findings have been reported. Even the more important anomalies discussed below are quite rare. The embryologic reasons for the variations relate in part to the development of the head and neck, which proceeds in very rapid and complex fashion during early embryogenesis. The cells that form many different facial structures lie close together, and a minimal stimulus may produce devastating consequences.

The most complex abnormalities, some of which have been discussed in other chapters, are those that have widespread effects on the normal development of the entire head and neck region. Facial clefts are the result of failure of fusion of facial mesoderm occurring at a very early stage of embryonic development. The most common example is a cleft lip or palate. The orbit is not often involved, and the only ocular manifestation may be a lower lid coloboma.

The facial dystrophies include abnormalities of the eye, facial structures, jaw and external and middle ear. All of these structures are derived from the first branchial arch and cleft. Because of this common origin and the relatively small area of involved tissue, numerous variations have been described. There is considerable overlap between different syndromes. Mandibulofacial dysostosis involves the lower face primarily, but colobomas of the lids are often seen. Goldenhar's syndrome (oculoauricular dysplasia) typically includes epibulbar dermoids, accessory auricular appendages, and aural fistulas. In addition, hypoplasia of the jaw, lid colobomas, and microphthalmia are associated with this syndrome. Patients with Hallermann-Streiff syndrome have a characteristic facial appearance, with mandibular hypoplasia, a sharp nose, microphthalmia, and secondary small orbits. These patients often show dwarfism and hypotrichosis.

A secondary group of congenital abnormalities affecting the orbit includes those that involve the skull. Premature closure of the sutures of the skull causes various bizarre skull shapes, including vertical elongation (oxycephaly), horizontal elongation (scaphocephaly), and other peculiar skull shapes. The abnormal sutural closure in many of these syndromes causes compression of the optic nerves and abnormalities in the formation of the orbit, with secondary proptosis or narrowing of the optic canal due to sphenoid bone hypoplasia. Optic atrophy may result. Somewhat similar findings are seen in the craniofacial dysostosis described by Crouzon. A more common orbital abnormality that shows a spectrum between minimal abnormality and marked abnormality is hypertelorism, in which there is wider separation of the eyes than normal. The size and bony construction of the orbits may be normal, but they are set at a much greater angle. The inverse abnormality, hypotelorism, is quite rare.[1]

The anomalies of cyclopia and synophthalmia are appropriate subjects for the transition between discussion of the diffuse facial abnormalities and discussion of those more strictly limited to the orbit. These rare abnormalities are probably related to abnormal function of the prosencephalic organizing center, which is responsible, among other things, for formation of the midfacial and orbital structures. Complete fusion of the two globes with total absence of the midline facial structures is properly called cyclopia. Still unusual, but more common, are partial fusions of the orbits and globes in varying degrees, referred to as synophthalmia. In addition to the ocular fusion, there is obviously abnormal orbital development, and there are varying degrees of deletion of portions of the anterior brain.

Minor variations in the bony composition of the orbital walls and in the locations of sutures, notches, and canals are common but are of little clinical significance. Complete absence of one or more of the bones forming the orbit wall is distinctly unusual. If the orbital roof is involved, there may be pulsating exophthalmos. Gross distortions of the orbit are often due to the sutural closure abnormalities previously mentioned.

Small openings in the orbit may allow orbital prolapse of portions of the meninges (meningocele) or brain tissue (encephalocele). These openings usually are found in the medial aspect of the orbit and may produce displacement or proptosis of the globe. Even though these abnormalities are unusual, the possibility of their existence should be borne in mind in the differential diagnosis of orbital masses in children.[1]

The association of microphthalmia with a congenital cyst of the orbit is an abnormality related to faulty closure of the choroidal fissure. This abnormality occurs between the third and sixth weeks of embryonic development. The globe is malformed, with abnormal anterior segment structures as well as partial or complete ocular colobomas associated with retinal and choroidal abnormalities. If the coloboma involves all ocular layers, a bulging cyst may develop behind the abnormal globe, causing extreme proptosis. Portions of retina, choroid, and abnormal mesodermal elements are found both within the eye and in the orbital cyst. The visual prognosis for such eyes is poor.[1,2] Congenital orbital tumors will be discussed later in this chapter.

In cases of severe microphthalmia or anophthalmia the extremely small or missing eye results in poor postnatal development of orbital structures. The absence or small size of the globe fails to provide a stimulus to orbital growth, which is similar to the situation seen when enucleation is necessary in early childhood. Complete absence of the eye is extremely unusual. In most cases, sectioning of the orbital reveals a small malformed globe or rudiments of various ocular structures. There is some tendency for inheritance of this condition. The genetic pattern is variable.

Lid abnormalities are more common than orbital abnormalities, but in most cases they present a less serious problem to the patient. Total absence of the lid structures is rare. Many varieties of congenital lid colobomas have been described. Usually the full thickness of the lid is missing in the involved area (Fig. 4–1). Attachment of the margins of the coloboma to the globe occurs. An abnormally large palpebral aperture is much less common than congenital blepharophimosis (Fig. 4–2), in which the palpebral opening is smaller than normal. This latter defect has a strong hereditary tendency, usually with an autosomal dominant pattern. Tilting of the palpebral aperture upward or downward is unusual. Congenital folds of lid skin may be a normal racial characteristic or may represent an isolated congenital anomaly. A semilunar fold of skin at the inner canthus extending from the upper lid to the lower lid is referred to as epicanthus (Fig. 4–3). This is a very common abnormality, and in most cases it disappears spontaneously with growth of the facial structures. Its principal clinical significance is that it may create the impression of esotropia when in fact none exists. Congenital entropion or ectropion are rare abnormalities (Figs. 4–4 and 4–5). The palpebral fissure may be shortened by fusion over part of its length, a condition known as ankyloblepharon. The outer canthal area is most commonly involved in this condition. Absence of the lashes is unusual. Extra rows of lashes (distichiasis) or an increase in the length of the lashes are common (Fig. 4–6). Usually, no treatment is indicated unless the lashes are in a position to rub against the cornea.[1] The problem of congenital ptosis was dealt with in an earlier chapter.

A congenital deficiency of lacrimal function is a rare anomaly that may be due to a variety of conditions, as discussed in the preceding chapter.

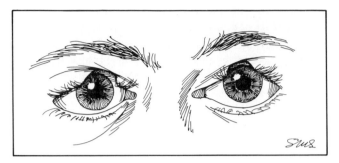

Figure 4-1.　Colobomas of both upper lids.

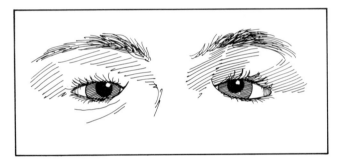

Figure 4-2.　Congenital blepharophimosis of both eyes.

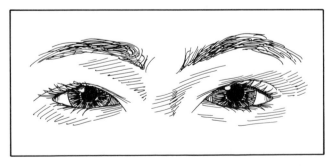

Figure 4-3.　Epicanthal folds.

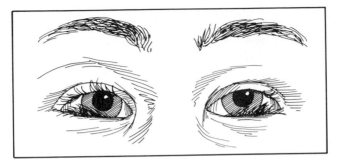

Figure 4-4. Entropion.

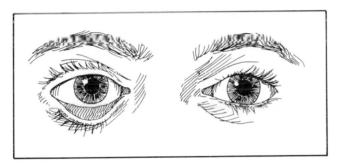

Figure 4-5. Ectropion of the right lower lid.

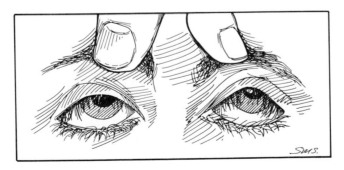

Figure 4-6. Distichiasis.

Aberrant lacrimal gland tissue may be found anywhere in the orbit or on the surface of the globe. It may be a cosmetic defect, or within the orbit it may produce proptosis. Congenital cysts or fistulas in the lacrimal gland area occur, but they are quite rare. Congenital obstruction of the lacrimal punctum and canaliculus is often seen. When there is obstruction to tear flow with persistent tearing, 70 percent of the time the obstruction is in the lacrimal duct. In many instances the lacrimal passages will open spontaneously. Expectant treatment for the first several months after birth is best, since probing of the lacrimal passages may result in structural damage that may make later surgery mandatory.[1]

INFLAMMATION

Of far greater importance than congenital orbital deformities are acute and chronic inflammatory diseases involving the orbit. Acute inflammation is of particularly serious import, not only because of the localized effects to the orbit and globe but also because of the danger of systemic spread, which often includes the central nervous system. Before discussing specific diseases, it may be useful to comment on some of the potential sources of infection. Inflammatory disease arising primarily in the orbit is uncommon. In most cases infection develops either from exogenous sources or by spread from neighboring areas. Penetrating injuries of the orbit are rare in children, but they do carry a risk of infection, particularly with a wood foreign body, which may carry dirt with bacteria or fungi deep into the orbit. The bone that separates the maxillary, sphenoid, and ethmoid sinuses from the orbit is thin and easily breached by infection. Spread of an infection from the paranasal sinuses used to be very common, but because of antibiotic therapy it is now less important. Direct spread from a dental infection is a rare possibility. Because of the anastomosis of the venous drainage of the periorbital area with the orbital veins, infections on the face and lids are frequently sources of organisms for orbital cellulitis. Spread of an infection from the globe or from intracranial infections also occurs, but it is quite unusual. Even less common are orbital infections arising from septicemia. Individuals with diabetes, leukemia, or other systemic disease are more prone to orbital inflammatory disease.

Regardless of the causative agent or source of infection, the clinical picture of orbital cellulitis presents a number of typical features that might be predicted from inflammation in this region. Because of the limited room in the orbit, proptosis occurs early and often is accompanied by lid swelling and conjunctival chemosis. Because of the inflammatory infiltrate, involvement of the extraocular muscles is common, and limitation of movement of the globe frequently is seen. Systemic effects of such infections depend on the nature of the infectious agent.

A number of complications of orbital cellulitis have serious consequences. Corneal ulceration due to exposure or direct involvement by the infectious agent may occur. Spread of the infection to involve the optic nerve can cause the development of papilledema and optic neuritis, with permanent visual loss. Severe proptosis may also accompany orbital cellulitis and may produce stretching of the optic nerve, with secondary atrophy. Involvement of the orbital venous drainage system can produce thrombophlebitis leading to cavernous sinus thrombosis. This, in turn, may spread elsewhere in the central nervous system. Even with adequate antibiotic therapy the mortality from cavernous sinus thrombosis is high. Because of the passage of various cranial nerves through the cavernous sinus, extraocular motor palsies and disturbance of function of the trigeminal nerve are common accompaniments of cavernous sinus disease. Bilateral involvement is often seen. Vigorous broad-spectrum antibiotic treatment and frequent neurological evaluation are most important in management of this condition.[1]

When infection spreads from one of the paranasal sinuses, involvement of the bone with osteomyelitis may occur. Proptosis may be a presenting sign. This disease is most often seen in children, and it may occur in the first few weeks of life. Most commonly, *staphylococcus* is the organism responsible. Specific antibiotic therapy is obviously important.

Chronic orbital inflammations, on the other hand, most often occur in adults. The proliferative aspect of chronic inflammation can result in the formation of an inflammatory pseudotumor of the orbit. This is a non-specific diagnosis, as indicated by the histopathologic findings, which may vary: proliferation of dense fibrous tissue; dense infiltrates of lymphocytes, plasma cells, and histiocytes; diffuse myositis involving all of the extraocular muscles. Computerized axial tomography often demonstrates enormous enlargement of the extraocular muscles. The etiology of this obviously diverse group of inflammatory responses is obscure.

Specific types of orbital inflammation, including those caused by common bacteria, are also encountered. At one time tuberculous and syphilitic orbital inflammations were important, but these are now rarely seen in children or adults. Orbital involvement with species of *Aspergillus* produces inflammatory orbital pseudotumor, although this is more common in adults than in children. On the other hand, infection caused by fungi belonging to the order Phycomycetes does occur in children and is important because of its potentially grave consequences. These organisms most frequently gain entry to the orbit through the paranasal sinuses and produce severe granulomatous orbital cellulitis that progresses with great rapidity. The ability of the organisms to invade normal orbital barriers may lead to endophthalmitis, cavernous sinus thrombosis, and diffuse intracranial involvement. Such infections may occur spontaneously in otherwise healthy patients. However, their highest incidence is in individuals with severe systemic disease, including childhood diabetes, renal failure, leukemia, chronic immunosuppression, or any systemic disease that produces severe debilitation. Phycomycosis often causes a typical orbital apex syndrome, with loss of vision, internal or external ophthalmoplegia, involvement of the fifth cranial nerve, or development of the Tolosa-Hunt syndrome. Gangrene of the central facial structures, including the nose and sinuses, is common. The development of disseminated cerebral infection with the organism frequently leads to a fatal outcome. Despite diffuse involvement of the paranasal sinuses, the presenting symptom may be rapid onset of proptosis and ophthalmoplegia. For this reason, prompt recognition of the possibility of this condition is most important to the pediatrician and ophthalmologist. Phycomycosis was at one time universally fatal; prompt diagnosis and treatment with systemic amphotericin B have resulted in survival of a number of patients. Other fungal organisms also may cause orbital inflammation, either by spread from the paranasal sinuses or by spread from an intracranial infection.[1,3-5]

In some parts of the world, parasitic infections of the orbit are seen in children. Trichinosis may affect children as well as adults, with acute onset of orbital cellulitis. Filariasis, echinococcosis, and cysticercosis also cause orbital disease in children. Myiasis occurs most often in undeveloped countries and may be accompanied by secondary bacterial infection.

LIDS

Contact dermatitis involving the lids occurs frequently and is caused by many different drugs and chemical agents. These include such things as atropine, antibiotics, and cosmetics. It may safely be stated that nearly any drug that comes in contact with the eye for a sufficient period of time is capable of producing contact dermatitis. Complaints include itching, redness, and breakdown of the skin due to rupture of vesicles. The primary treatment is removal of the etiologic agent, if possible. Systemic antihistamine preparations and topical corticosteroids provide symptomatic relief.

In addition to contact allergies, systemic medications may produce cutaneous responses that involve the eyes. Antibiotics, barbiturates, and heavy metals such as arsenic and gold can cause allergic dermatitis.

Many infectious agents are capable of producing local or diffuse lid inflammation. This can present in many ways, including localized abscesses or impetiginous reactions. In rare instances infectious bullous impetigo may progress to generalized exfoliative dermatitis. In infants this syndrome is referred to as Ritter's disease. In older children a similar clinical picture is called toxic epidermal necrolysis (Lyell's disease). Streptococcal infections are particularly prone to cause erysipeloid inflammation involving not only the lids but also large areas of the face. Gram stain, cultures, and appropriate antibiotic therapy are indicated in all forms of infectious lid conditions. Congenital syphilis seldom affects the lids in children, but it may produce ulceration at the outer canthus. Primary lesions of syphilis are rarely seen.[1]

Viral infections of the lid may be produced by vaccinia virus and may consist of multiple pustules that produce scarring or orbital cellulitis. Herpes simplex also appears in its primary form on the lids, although corneal involvement is far more serious. Idoxuridine is of questionable value for cutaneous herpes. Vidarabine ointment may be useful. Varicella may affect the lids and produce considerable swelling, but serious consequences are unusual. The related zoster virus is generally a disease of adults, but it may occur in infants and children as well. If the nasociliary branch of the fifth nerve is involved, the possibility of lid and intraocular inflammation exists. This virus can cause devastating keratouveitis, with secondary glaucoma, cataract, and posterior pole inflammation. Any child with a zoster infection should be seen promptly by an ophthalmologist and should be followed carefully for the duration of the active disease.

The virus that produces verrucae can involve the lids as well as other parts of the body. It is often spread by autoinoculation and may produce multiple lesions arranged in linear fashion. On occasion the keratin flakes produced from the verrucae may fall into the conjunctival sac and cause mild keratitis. Probably the safest method of treatment is freezing with solid carbon dioxide or liquid nitrogen. Use of chemical cauterization around the eyes should be done with extreme care because of possible corneal consequences.

Another viral infection commonly seen in children is molluscum contagiosum. This disease is characterized by elevated umbilicated lesions on the upper or lower lids. There may be resistant low-grade keratoconjunctivitis that is best treated by excision of the molluscum lesions.

Fungal lid infections involve many types of organisms. Adults are involved more frequently than children. Children with disseminated *Candida* infections may have eyelid involvement. *Tinea* and *Trichophyton* may spread to the eye from other parts of the body. Generally lid involvement is unusual.[1]

Parasitic infections that affect the lids include filariasis, onchocerciasis, and schistosomiasis in endemic areas. A much more common parasitic disease as far as children are concerned is pediculosis, which produces symptoms similar to those seen elsewhere in the body with this arthropod. The crab louse (*Phthirus*) may also infest the lids and lashes. Mechanical removal or application of 1 percent physostigmine or gama benzene hexachloride ointment is quite effective.

The name blepharitis refers to acute or chronic inflammation of the lid margin. This may be accompanied by ulceration or thickening fo the lids, as well as dryness or scaling. *Staphylococcus* is often the infectious agent. Individuals with seborrhea are particularly likely to develop this condition. Daily cleaning of the lid margins to remove all scales and exudative debris is probably the most important treatment. This can be supplemented by application of an antibiotic-steroid ointment to the lid margins to eliminate the staphylococci and decrease the inflammatory reaction. This is one of the rare instances in which this drug combination is indicated.

Without question the most common inflammatory disease of the lids is the stye. This is caused by staphylococcal infection of a hair follicle. Multiple sties can cause considerable edema and pain. Although sties usually resolve with conservative measures, including warm soaks and topical antibiotics, the potential for orbital cellulitis and its complications should be kept in mind. A stye often is followed by a chalazion, which is a chronic inflammatory reaction involving a sebaceous gland of the lid. Chalazions may be most prominent externally, or they may present on the tarsal conjunctival surface. They are firm, well circumscribed, and usually freely movable. Often they will disappear spontaneously after several months, but if they present cosmetic defects, they can easily be removed by simple surgical procedures.

Acute inflammations of the lacrimal gland (dacryoadenitis) are rare in both children and adults. Such inflammations may be due to spread of preexisting inflammatory disease from elsewhere on the face. In children the most common cause is lacrimal gland involvement by mumps virus. The lacrimal gland may be involved in sarcoidosis, but such involvement is very rare. Disease of the lacrimal canaliculi is unusual; it is perhaps most commonly caused by infection with species of *Actinomyces*. This is usually a unilateral disease characterized by tearing, despite apparently normal passage of fluid on irrigation of the lacrimal drainage system. Patients often have persistent conjunctivitis. A suggestive clue is enlargement of the lacrimal punctum. The proliferative masses of fungal organisms must be curetted from the lacrimal passages. Acute and chronic dacryocystitis is a fairly common disease associated with obstruction of the lacrimal drainage system and is caused by a variety of bacterial organisms. Severe and painful swelling, with discharge from the lacrimal punctum, is evident. Massage over the lacrimal sac will express purulent material. Severe acute dacryocystitis may drain spontaneously through the skin below the inner canthus, causing establishment of a permanent fistula. The severity of the inflammation and the scar tissue it produces often result in permanent obstruction of the lacrimal drainage channels. Dacryocystorhinostomy is needed in such cases to cure the tearing problem.

TUMORS

Because of the many different types of epithelial and mesodermal tissue found in the normal orbit, it is not surprising that many varieties of benign and malignant tumors originate in this location. Taken individually, an orbital tumor of any type is quite rare in the pediatric age group. In fact, orbital tumors in general are far from being common ophthalmological problems. In a review of over 100 orbital tumors[6] it was found that about 20 percent of the tumors occurred in patients under 15 years of age. Because of the many varieties of histologic types that are found, the differential diagnosis is quite difficult. It is not particularly helpful to look at tables of incidence, because the frequencies in any particular study depend on the bias of the particular collection. For example, Porterfield's study is heavily weighted in favor of rhabdomyosarcoma, as well as tumors of the optic nerve (Table 4–1). Each of these tumors, although important, is certainly many times less common than hemangioma of the orbit. In Porterfield's series only three metastatic tumors were found, all of them neuroblastomas.[6] This relatively common malignancy of children obviously should have a much higher incidence. Because of the tendency to submit unusual tumors and diagnostic problems to the Armed Forces Institute of Pathology, the table is more important from the viewpoint of considering diagnostic possibilities than as an indication of relative frequencies of occurrence.

The clinical signs found in patients with orbital tumors include proptosis, swelling of the orbital tissues, and changes in ocular motility. If the tumor is pressing on the globe from any direction, changes in refraction may be pro-

Table 4–1
Orbital Tumors (214) in Children*

Primary nonepithelial	71
Malignant 65 (56 rhabdomyosarcoma)	
Benign 6	
Optic nerve and meninges	39
Hamartomas (28 vascular)	35
Choristomas (17 dermoid)	18
Pseudotumors (10 inflammatory)	18
Lymphoma/leukemia	12
Unclassified malignancy	11
Lacrimal gland (3 adenocarcinoma)	4
Metastatic neuroblastoma	3
Microphthalmia with cyst	3

*Adapted from Porterfield.[6]

gressive. A tumor located near the posterior wall of the globe often indents the posterior pole and produces retinal folds that are easily seen with the ophthalmoscope. If the orbital blood supply is involved, especially the venous drainage, the anterior segment may show hyperemia. A slow rate of growth often but not always suggests a benign tumor, whereas rapid growth sways the differential diagnosis in the direction of malignancy. The tumor may grow in any direction, although some tumors have a propensity for producing directional proptosis. For example, a dermoid usually pushes the eye in an inferonasal direction. Too much diagnostic importance should not be attached to the direction of proptosis.

A variety of diagnostic procedures may be helpful, including standard x-rays, computerized axial tomography, ultrasound examination, arteriograms, and venograms. A careful history and examination are often the best means of directing diagnostic suspicions. For example, an individual with multiple café au lait spots may have neurofibromatosis. Such patients have increased incidences of glioma of the optic nerve. In many cases a definitive diagnosis cannot be made by clinical and laboratory examination, and orbital exploration with diagnostic biopsy is necessary. Because of the danger of injury to orbital structures during surgical exploration, this should not be undertaken until all diagnostic approaches are completed.

Dermoid and epidermoid cysts are the most common choristomas found in the orbit, particularly in the pediatric age group. Dermoids present as painless swellings, often along the upper temporal orbital margin. Because of the slow development of the tumor, it may not make its first clinical appearance until adult life. In some cases the tumor is attached to the bony wall of the orbit, but this does not indicate malignant change. When the orbital wall is involved, characteristic x-ray changes are seen. Neither dermoid cysts nor epidermoid cysts have malignant potential. They produce their symptoms chiefly by virtue of their size and pressure on adjacent structures. Because the contents of the cyst may be oily, care should be taken during surgical removal. A cyst that ruptures during surgery or after trauma and releases its contents into the orbit can cause a marked granulomatous inflammatory reaction. The other choristomas that occur in the orbit are less common; they include teratoma and ectopic lacrimal gland. Orbital teratomas appear during the neonatal period; they may be composed of all tissue layers and may contain differential structures from multiple organs. Ectopic lacrimal gland may produce proptosis if there is a sufficient mass. Its appearance is identical with that of normal lacrimal gland, and such deposits have no malignant potential.[1]

Tumors composed of vascular tissue are probably the most common primary orbital neoplasms in children. Although there are several varieties, capillary and cavernous hemangiomas of the orbit are most often seen. Capillary hemangiomas usually appear during the first 5 years of life; as with cutaneous hemangiomas, they frequently show spontaneous regression. For this reason, if the diagnosis is certain, surgical intervention should be avoided. A cavernous hemangioma often has a well-defined capsule and frequently is located within the muscle cone. Because of this location, in addition to producing proptosis, it may produce retinal folds and changes in refraction due to direct pressure on the globe. Proptosis increases in situations that produce an increase in venous pressure, such as crying or straining. Conversely, firm gentle pressure applied over the orbit will temporarily reduce the proptosis as blood is drained from the hemangioma. Lymphangioma also usually presents in young children and shows spontaneous regression. Hemorrhage into the stroma of a lymphangioma may make histopathologic differentiation from hemangioma difficult. Hemangioendothelioma is most common during the first few months of life; about 20 percent are evident at birth. This tumor consists of a proliferation of endothelial cells and contains very few passages for circulating blood. Arteriovenous malformations in the orbit are unusual, but they may produce intermittent attacks of painful proptosis. Because of the diffuse nature of the malformation, treatment is extremely difficult. Malignant orbital vascular tumor may occur, but it is a disease of adults rather than of children.

Although all orbital tumors are uncommon, rhabdomyosarcoma is generally considered to be the most common primary malignant neoplasm of the orbit (excluding the globe) in children. The majority of patients are younger than 10 years of age. This tumor does not occur exclusively in the orbit, but the orbit is a common site for it. Growth of the tumor is often rapid, and proptosis is striking. In the early stages the proptosis tends to be in an inferotemporal direction. The tumor does not arise from the extraocular muscles but from undifferentiated mesenchymal tissues of the orbit. Several histopathologic varieties of rhabdomyosarcoma are seen. These include the differentiated variety, in which the tumor cells show typical features of striated muscle. Most common is the embryonal form, in which mitotic activity is abundant and no differentiation is evident. Most unusual is the alveolar type, which has a pseudoglandular appearance. Rhabdomyosarcoma is associated with a high mortality rate ranging between 40 and 60 percent. Without treatment the survival rate is virtually zero. Orbital exenteration and radiation were originally the treatments of choice. Recently, some success has been achieved with radiation alone.[3,4,7]

Although glioma arises from the optic nerve rather than from orbital tissue, it is appropriate to consider glioma here. This is a relatively common tumor, and over 85 percent are seen in patients under 15 years of age. Girls outnumber boys by a ratio of about 2:1. Proptosis is usually in the straightforward direction. Visual acuity often is decreased early in the development of the tumor. The classic x-ray sign is enlargement of the optic foramen, but this may be difficult to demonstrate without excellent radiology facilities. Furthermore, a tumor adjacent to the globe can grow to large size without involving the optic foramen. Therefore, absence of this x-ray finding does not rule out the diagnosis. In any patient in whom this tumor is suspected as part of the differential diagnosis, a careful review of family history and a careful examination of the patient for signs of neurofibromatosis are indicated, since gliomas of the optic nerve occur frequently in this syndrome. Neurofibromatosis is discussed in greater detail in the section on the phakomatoses. Gliomas do not produce distant metastases, but in their growth backward along the optic nerve they eventually involve the optic foramen and the intracranial portions of the optic nerve. Extension may include the optic chiasm. Meningioma involving the orbit in children is less common than it is in adults.[3,4,7]

Discussion of orbital tumors, including lymphoma, leukemia, and allied disorders, is complicated by the geographic variation in incidence and the relative infrequency with which many of these tumors are seen by ophthalmologists. In Africa, for instance, Burkitt's lymphoma is a common cause of orbital disease. In a series of orbital tumors in African children[8] almost 50 percent of the diagnosed disease was due to Burkitt's lymphoma. Even when considering orbital tumors without regard to age group,[9] this tumor made up nearly 30 percent of the total number of orbital tumors. Whereas this tumor is common in Africa, it is less so in the United States, but it has been reported with both orbital and intraocular involvement.[10] Both lymphoma and leukemia may involve the orbit, most typically late in the disease. Acute myeloblastic leukemia may have its primary presentation in the orbit. This is another lesion that is particularly common in Africa. Hodgkin's disease rarely affects the orbit. In most instances of lymphoma and leukemia the diagnosis is already apparent, and the orbital problem is a secondary manifestation.

Inflammatory pseudotumors of the orbit are common in adults but less so in children. As previously discussed, these may show a variety of inflammatory patterns, including myositis, fibrosis, or a dense infiltrate of lymphocytes and plasma cells. They may be related to disease of adjacent structures, or they may appear as a primary finding. The reactive type of lymphoid or plasma cell hyperplasia has often been mistaken in the past for primary orbital lymphoma. Careful examination of the histopathology reveals a polymorphic infiltrate that is helpful in differentiation. Reactive lymphoid hyperplasia may be associated with abnormal serum proteins (e.g., macroglobulinemia).[3,4,7]

Diseases included under the nonspecific name Histiocytosis X include eosinophilic granuloma, Hand-Schüller-Christian disease, and Letterer-Siwe disease, all of which may affect the orbits. Eosinophilic granuloma often involves the orbital rim, and pathologic examination of an affected area shows the characteristic histiocytes combined with an infiltrate of eosinophils. The classic findings of Hand-Schüller-Christian disease include multiple bony skull lesions, diabetes insipidus, and exophthalmos. The exophthalmos is produced by diffuse histiocytic infiltration of the orbit. Juvenile xanthogranuloma is sometimes considered as one of the histiocytoses, but its relationship to the other disorders remains unclear. Orbital involvement in this disease is nowhere near as common as cutaneous involvement or intraocular involvement, which are discussed elsewhere.[3,4,7,11]

Metastatic orbital tumors are rarely seen in the eye pathology laboratory, but clinically they are much more common. Orbital metastatic disease is typically a terminal event, and the diagnosis is usually apparent. In the pediatric age group neuroblastoma is by far the most common metastatic orbital lesion. Orbital involvement by lymphoma and leukemia has already been discussed. Orbital extension of a retinoblastoma is a common mode of local spread, although the tumor itself is rare.

The syndromes characterized by the development of hamartomas involving multiple organ syndromes are referred to as the phakomatoses. These syndromes classically include angiomatosis retinae (von Hippel's disease), neurofibromatosis (von Recklinghausen's disease), tuberous sclerosis (Bourneville's syndrome), Sturge-Weber syndrome, ataxia-telangiectasia (Louis-Bar syndrome), and Wyburn-Mason syndrome. Only neurofibromatosis has important orbital effects. Involvement of the lids with plexiform neurofibromas may produce severe distortion. In addition, these may affect the orbital roof, producing a defect associated with pulsating exophthalmos. The high incidence of gliomas of the optic nerve in patients with this syndrome has already been mentioned. There is also an increase in the frequency of meningiomas. Possibly related to neurofibromatosis is the syndrome characterized by medullary carcinoma of the thyroid, pheochromocytoma, and multiple mucosal neuromas. As far as the eyes are concerned, the medullary carcinoma syndrome can cause thickening of the lid margins, alterations in placement of the lashes, and thickening of the corneal nerves. The other phakomatoses produce no significant orbital involvement. Ataxia-telangiectasia is associated with conjunctival vascular abnormalities. The lesions of tuberous sclerosis may involve the eyelids. The cutaneous angiomas of the Sturge-Weber syndrome that may involve the eyelids are well known.[3,4,12]

In adults the wide variety of lid lesions can produce many problems in differential diagnosis. The clinical possibilities are more limited in children. Primary lid malignancies are extremely rare in children, and many of the degenerative lesions associated with age and solar exposure, such as senile keratosis, need not be considered here.

A lid lesion common to both children and adults is papilloma. This is really a descriptive name rather than a specific diagnosis; it refers to thickening and folding of the layers of the epidermis. As is the case with the conjunctiva, some papillomas have a viral origin and may be multiple. A variety of clinical appearances can be seen, including both flat and elevated pedunculated lesions. Simple excision is appropriate treatment if a cosmetic defect exists. Sebaceous and epidermoid cysts are seen in the lids; these are usually well-circumscribed, freely movable lesions that do not exhibit growth.

In adults, basal cell epithelioma is the most common primary malignant lid tumor, whereas squamous cell carcinoma is extremely rare. Both of these lesions are rare in children, except for those individuals afflicted with the recessively inherited disease known as xeroderma pigmentosum. Such patients have a marked sensitivity to sunlight; following months or years of exposure, they develop focal pigmentary changes, atrophy, and telangiectasia of the skin suggesting radiation exposure. In many patients with this syndrome, including those in the pediatric age group, multiple neoplasms appear, including squamous cell carcinoma, basal cell carcinoma, and malignant melanoma. Multicentric and diffuse involvement of the skin make this disease difficult to treat.[3,4]

Benign pigmented lesions of varying histology are commonly seen in children. Ephelis or freckle is a benign lesion characterized by increased pigment in the basal layer of the epithelium. Both the histologic classification and the clinical appearance of pigmented nevi often causes diagnostic confusion. The clinical presentation may be of a flat, elevated, pedunculated papillomatous or hairy lesions. Although pigmentation is often associated with nevi, many are completely amelanotic. There are three important histologic types of nevi: (1) junctional, in which nevus cells are located in the deep layers of the epidermis, and little or no dermal involvement is seen; (2) intradermal, in which the nevus cells are isolated in the dermis, and the lesion is often amelanotic; (3) compound, in which features of both junctional and intradermal nevi are present. Dermal nevi rarely give rise to malignant melanoma. Junctional nevi are the most likely precursors of malignant melanoma, and compound nevi are intermediate. Malignant melanoma arising in the lids is extremely uncommon in children.[3,4,7]

Because of the complicated histology of the lids, it is not surprising that a wide variety of other tumors occur. Tumors of blood vessels, including hemangiomas, lymphangiomas, and hemangioendotheliomas, are seen in young individuals. On occasion, capillary or cavernous hemangiomas may cause marked cosmetic defects. Characteristically these are not too prominent at birth, but within a few weeks they show alarming growth. Various therapeutic maneuvers have been attempted with hemangiomas, including surgery and injection of sclerosing solutions. Both treatment alternatives often result in permanent scarring and functional loss as far as the lid is concerned.

In the overwhelming majority of cases, parents should be advised to wait until the child is at least 2–3 years old before considering the possibility of surgery. The most frequent clinical course is that the hemangioma begins to atrophy with time, and it may spontaneously disappear with minimal or no cosmetic defect. This, of course, is not true in the Sturge-Weber syndrome.[3,4,7]

Inflammatory lesions of the lacrimal system have already been discussed; they are the most common cause of swelling involving the lacrimal gland or lacrimal drainage system. Epithelial tumors of the lacrimal drainage system are rare and are limited to adults. Inflammatory pseudotumors may involve the lacrimal gland or may appear in the orbit, as previously discussed.

Systemic disease involving the orbit in children is relatively uncommon. In the rare cases of involvement with one of the collagen diseases in children, orbital manifestations may be seen. The syndromes known variously as allergic vasculitis, Wegener's granulomatosis, and lethal midline granuloma may all be related to periarteritis nodosa. All such lesions are characterized by granulomatous periarteritis. Both lids and orbit may be involved by these inflammatory lesions, and lupus erythematosus may cause inflammatory orbital pseudotumor or arteritis, but this is uncommon in children. Dermatomyositis may begin in childhood with exophalmos and paralysis of the extraocular muscles.

Endocrine exophthalmos presents a severe ophthalmic problem in adults, but it is rarely seen in children. In those unusual instances in which it may enter into differential diagnosis, it should be kept in mind that the eye signs are often asymmetric. It is well known that in adults endocrine exophthalmos is the most common cause of unilateral exophthalmos. Whereas this is certainly not true in children, the possibility should always be considered.

Sarcoidosis is not common in children, but when it occurs there may be involvement of the retina, optic nerve, orbit, lacrimal gland, and lid skin with characteristic noncaseating granulomas. Uveitis and retinal periphlebitis are discussed elsewhere.[1]

REFERENCES

1. Duke-Elder S: System of Ophthalmology, vol XIII, The Ocular Adnexa. London, Henry Kimpton, 1974
2. Makley TA, Battles M: Microphthalmos with cyst. Surv Ophthalmol 13:200, 1969
3. Hogan MJ, Zimmerman LE: Ophthalmic Pathology. Philadelphia, WB Saunders, 1962
4. Yanoff M, Fine BS: Ocular Pathology. New York, Harper & Row, 1975
5. Blodi FC, Hannah FT, Wadsworth JAC: Lethal orbital-cerebral phycomycosis: In otherwise healthy children. Am J Ophthalmol 67:698, 1969

6. Porterfield, JF: Orbital tumors in children: A report on 214 cases. Int Ophthalmol Clin 2:319, 1962
7. Reese AB: Tumors of the Eye (ed 3). New York, Harper & Row, 1976
8. Templeton AC: Orbital tumors in African children. Br J Ophthalmol 55:254, 1971
9. Olurin O, Williams A: Orbital-ocular tumors in Nigeria. Cancer 30:580, 1972
10. Feman SS, Niwayama G, Hepler RS, Foos RY: Burkitt tumor with intraocular involvement. Surv Ophthalmol 14:106, 1969
11. Codling BW, Soni KC, Barry DR, Martin-Walker W: Histocytosis presenting as swelling of orbit and eyelid. Br J Ophthalmol 56:517, 1972
12. Font RL, Ferry AP: The phakomatoses. Int Ophthalmal Clin 12:1, 1972

Pei-Fei Lee, M.D.

5
Congenital Glaucoma

Glaucoma may be defined as any eye disease characterized by abnormally high intraocular pressure that results in either temporary or permanent impairment of visual function or optic nerve conductivity. Glaucoma has been classified into two broad categories: primary glaucomas and secondary glaucomas. It has been further divided into three groups according to the age of the patient: congenital (infantile), juvenile, and adult. Glaucoma is called primary when it is unrelated to other eye disease or abnormalities; it is secondary when it develops as a consequence of eye disease or developmental abnormalities.

Congenital glaucoma has been defined by Chandler and Scheie as glaucoma occurring in individuals under 30 years of age; it is divided into infantile and juvenile types. It is referred to as infantile glaucoma when it occurs between the time of birth and 5 years of age; juvenile glaucoma refers to glaucoma developed between the ages of 6 and 30 years. Congenital glaucoma is a very serious but relatively uncommon eye disease among infants and children. Therefore it is not unusual to see an untreated case of far-advanced congenital glaucoma that was neglected by the patient's family and physicians as well; much of the useful vision could have been preserved if only it had been recognized early and appropriately treated in time. Early recognition by parents, obstetricians, pediatricians, psychiatrists, and ophthalmologists is essential in the successful management of congenital glaucoma and the prevention of blindness.

A brief description of congenital glaucoma, infantile and juvenile, is given in Table 5–1 and Table 5–2. Details are described in the text and in the appropriate sources.[1-5]

Table 5–1
Congenital (Infantile) Glaucoma

Features
  Eighty percent bilateral; 65% are males. In 80–90% the onset is within the first
    year of life (about 30% present at birth, 60% at 6 months, and 90% by end of
    first year). Autosomal recessive inheritance.

Symptoms and signs
  (1) Epiphora, photophobia, blepharospasm; (2) corneal edema and enlargement;
    (3) increased intraocular pressure; (4) ruptures (tears) in Descemet's membrane;
    (5) extension of physiologic cupping and atrophy of disk; (6) PMR

Probable causes or pathogenesis
  (1) Impermeable membrane; (2) abnormal iris insertion; (3) insertion of longitudi-
    nal ciliary muscle fibers into corneoscleral meshwork; (4) malformation of vas-
    cular system of eye; (5) inborn metabolic error

  Other conditions that may involve congenital abnormalities of filtration angle and
    congenital glaucoma: (1) late congenital or infantile glaucoma; (2) aniridia; (3)
    Sturge-Weber syndrome; (4) neurofibromatosis; (5) Marfan's syndrome; (6)
    Rieger's anomaly; (7) Peter's anomaly; (8) Lowe's syndrome; (9) Pierre Robin
    syndrome; (10) rubella syndrome

  Conditions with congenitally normal filtration angle and occasional congenital
    glaucoma: (1) persistent hyperplastic primary vitreous; (2) microcornea; (3) re-
    tinoblastoma; (4) retrolental fibroplasia; (5) homocystinuria; (6) spherophakia;
    (7) juvenile xanthogranuloma; (8) trisomy 18; (9) uveitis, dermatitis; (10)
    trauma; (11) steroid-induced glaucoma

  Conditions to be differentiated from congenital glaucoma: (1) megalocornea; (2)
    forceps injury; (3) keratitis; (4) mucopolysaccharidosis; (5) cystinosis; (6) con-
    genital hereditary corneal dystrophy; (7) inpatent nasolacrimal duct

Associated anomalies
  Numerous ocular and systemic anomalies may be associated with congenital
    glaucoma. Patients with anomalies listed below should be carefully evaluated
    for glaucoma because it may begin at any time in life.

Ocular anomalies
  (1) Iridocorneal dysgenesis (anterior chamber cleavage syndrome), (a) posterior
    embryotoxin of Axenfeld, (b) Rieger's syndrome; (2) essential iris atrophy; (3)
    aniridia; (4) pigmentary glaucoma; (5) megalocornea; (6) microcornea; (7) mic-
    rophthalmia; (8) spherophakia (microphakia); (9) myopia; (10) retinitis pigmen-
    tosa; (11) spontaneous hyphema; (12) glaucoma secondary to local ocular dis-
    ease

Treatment
  (1) Goniotomy—closed, open sky (direct); (2) trabeculotomy ab externo; (3) filtra-
    tion procedures, or other new glaucoma surgical procedures when goniotomy or
    trabeculotomy fails to control ocular tension; (4) cyclocryotherapy, when other
    procedures fail; (5) frequent examinations under general anesthesia; (6) total
    child care

Table 5–1 (continued)

Continuous care and prognosis
(1) Short-term; (2) long-term postoperative follow-up care

INFANTILE GLAUCOMA

Approximately 80 percent of patients have bilateral disorders; 65 percent of such patients are males. In 80–90 percent of cases the onset is within the first year of life (about 30 percent at birth, 60 percent at 6 months of age, and 90 percent by the end of the first year). It is generally considered as an autosomal recessive variety.

Buphthalmia, a prominent feature of infantile glaucoma, usually develops when glaucoma occurs at birth or early in life. This occurs because the sclera and cornea in infant eyes are unable to withstand sustained elevations in intraocular pressure. No appreciable enlargement of the eyes is expected when glaucoma develops after 1–2 years of age.

Table 5–2
Juvenile (Late Congenital) Glaucoma

Age & sex: Between 6 and 30 years of age; occurs most often in males.
Refraction & visual acuity: 83% myopic; that is why most juvenile glaucoma is recognized at the time of refraction.
History: Strong family history of open-angle glaucoma (about 20%). Incidence is about 0.01% at Wills Eye Hospital.
Cornea: Normal size, maybe even smaller than normal. No juvenile glaucoma eyes have large cornea or buphthalmos.
Intraocular pressure: Moderate to high pressure, usually in the range of 30–40 mm Hg.
Optic disk: Usually, long-standing pressure elevation and hence marked cupping and atrophy are common, frequently associated with visual field changes.
Symptoms: Poor vision; referred by school nurse for eye examination. It is the usual presenting symptom. Visual field defect is not uncommon at initial visit.
Treatment: More difficult to treat successfully than other types of glaucoma. Responds very poorly to treatment, and should be followed indefinitely.
Medication: Same as for an adult.
Surgery: Cases with early onset do better with goniotomy; cases with late onset do better with trabeculotomy or trabeculectomy.
Follow-up: Indefinitely; optic disk examination and visual fields are most helpful. Pressure variation and difficulties in follow-up.

Incidence

The incidence of infantile glaucoma is much lower than that of glaucoma in older individuals. No accurate figures for incidence of congenital glaucoma in the general population are available. In the statistics available from various glaucoma clinics, the incidence varies from 0.03 to 0.079 percent; it was 0.011 percent among 250,000 patients at the Wills Eye Hospital.[7] Generally, an ophthalmologist may encounter 1 case during a period of 5–10 years. Of the infants affected, 65 percent are males; glaucoma is bilateral in approximately 80 percent. Infantile glaucoma accounts for 5–13 percent of blindness among persons in schools for the blind,[8] much of which could have been prevented by early diagnosis and proper management.

Probable Causes of Pathogenesis

Congenital glaucoma induced by developmental abnormalities in the anterior chamber angle and ocular structures may be related to the following factors:

1. Impermeable membrane within the anterior chamber angle
2. Abnormal iris insertion
3. Insertion of longitudinal ciliary muscle fibers into the corneoscleral meshwork
4. Malformation of vascular system of the eye
5. Inborn metabolic errors
6. Injuries
7. Inflammation and infection
8. Others

Symptoms and Signs

Generally, regardless of the causes for increased intraocular pressure, the signs and symptoms of congenital glaucoma are quite similar at birth and during infancy and early childhood; they should be readily recognized by pediatricians and primary care physicians. Infants with glaucoma tend to be fussy and have poor eating habits; they have tearing and photophobia, and they frequently rub their eyes. Clinically, classic signs and symptoms of infantile glaucoma are as follows:

1. Epiphora, photophobia, blepharospasm
2. Corneal edema and enlargement of the cornea
3. Increased intraocular pressure
4. Ruptures (tears) in Descemet's membrane
5. Extension of the physiologic cupping and atrophy of the optic disk
6. Pseudo mental retardation

Tearing (epiphora), photophobia, and blepharospasm are three of the early and most common symptoms of infantile glaucoma that call the condition to the attention of the parents and pediatrician. Whenever unexplained tearing and photophobia are present in an infant or during the first 2 years of life, infantile glaucoma should always be suspected and excluded. Another cause of tearing in infants is obstruction of the tear ducts in the first year of life; however, there is no photophobia, and this tearing is not associated with corneal haze or buphthalmos. Tearing and photophobia likely result from corneal edema and mechanical irritations. This is the reason infants with congenital glaucoma seem to prefer darker environments and surroundings; they also may keep their eyes closed or bend over the parent's shoulder when exposed to bright surroundings, especially under bright sun. They may not wish to play outside of the house, preferring to be left alone in a darker room. Abnormal behavior may develop because of the tearing and photophobia that make the infant unhappy and uncooperative (Fig. 5–1). These symptoms are reversible once glaucoma is arrested or is under adequate control and stabilized.

Corneal edema and enlargement are usually presenting signs of established infantile glaucoma that may call the condition to the attention of parents because the infant or child experiences visual difficulties. Corneal haze is usually due to epithelial and subepithelial edema at the initial stage. It may progress and may even involve corneal stroma with complete corneal opacity

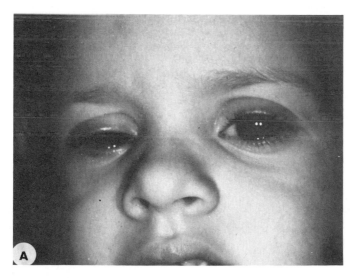

Figure 5–1A.   Tearing and photophobia in a 2-year-old child with far-advanced infantile glaucoma.

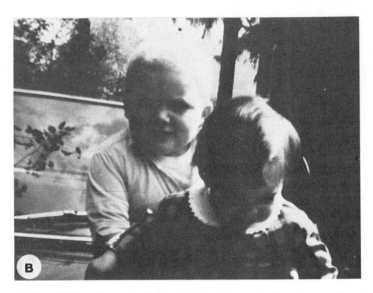

Figure 5–1B. Child with marked photophobia who cried when she was brought into bright sun. The opposite was true of her brother, who enjoyed sunlight. This 18-month-old girl had bilateral infantile glaucoma.

resembling modified scleral tissue or ground glass, especially at the limbal area.

If glaucoma is untreated, corneal size enlarges progressively until the corneal diameter reaches an obvious abnormal size or a buphthalmic state associated with further increase in corneal edema develops. Until 1 year of age the infant eye is very elastic, and if intraocular pressure builds up, the eye becomes larger, producing buphthalmos. However, when glaucoma develops after the age of 1 year, buphthalmos is less likely to occur.

Repeated corneal diameter measurement is important in the diagnosis and follow-up. An infant with corneal horizontal diameter greater than 12 mm or a cornea that is increasing in size should be considered and treated as an infantile glaucoma suspect until proven otherwise (Fig. 5–2).

Corneal thinning and stretching takes place at the limbal area, and continuing enlargement of the cornea may lead to rupture in Descemet's membrane, which is less elastic and is under constant tension. The ruptures may be linear, horizontal, branching, multiple, or single. It can cause localized or generalized corneal edema if aqueous diffuses into the corneal stroma along the course of the ruptures. The corneal edema clears when intraocular pressure is normalized, but the ruptures in Descemet's membrane remain visible permanently.

It should be kept in mind that corneal haze and ruptures in Descemet's

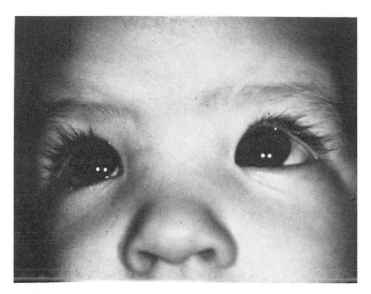

Figure 5–2.   Unilateral infantile glaucoma (O.S.) in 14-month-old infant. Corneal diameters were 11.5 mm O.D. and 14 mm O.S., associated with mild corneal edema and multiple linear ruptures in Descemet's membrane. Intraocular pressure under anesthesia was 7 mm Hg O.D. and 24 mm Hg O.S. This photograph was taken 1 year after successful surgery. Symptoms of tearing and photophobia have disappeared, and cornea is clear. Ruptures in Descemet's membrane are still visible with ophthalmoscope or with slit-lamp biomicroscope. There was no reverse of the corneal diameter despite the successful operation.

membrane can also be seen in infants as a result of birth injury. However, these are usually unilaterlal, and the intraocular pressure is normal. In addition, corneal haze can occur in a number of inborn errors and/or metabolic disorders, as well as other systemic conditions that are discussed elsewhere.

An intraocular pressure measurement and a detailed eye examination under general anesthesia are necessary to establish the diagnosis of infantile glaucoma and to exclude the other abnormalities or ocular pathology. Intraocular pressure is measured with portable applanation (Draeger or Perkins) or indentation (Schiøtz) tonometers. As in juvenile glaucoma, significant fluctuation or diurnal variation in intraocular pressure can occur and can cause erroneous tonometer readings. Therefore, other parameters or objective signs of infantile glaucoma must be used in the final diagnosis and in evaluating appropriate treatment. Tonography is of less value in the diagnosis and follow-up care of patients with infantile and juvenile glaucomas than in those with adult glaucomas. The technique is difficult to perform properly in children, and the results obtained in an anesthetized infant or child are uncertain.

The levels of intraocular pressure in normal children and in children with infantile glaucoma under general anesthesia are given in Table 5–3. The actual mean values for intraocular pressure are somewhat lower than those for adults. Generally, intraocular pressure is measured as part of a detailed eye examination under anesthesia.

Radtke and Cohan[12] recently reported that intraocular pressure can be measured satisfactorily with topical anesthesia in newborns. The average value of intraocular pressure in 60 awake and unrestrained full-term newborn infants was 11.4 ± 2.4 mm Hg, with the upper limits of normal being 17 mm Hg using the Perkins hand-held applanation tonometer. These values, obtained under topical anesthesia in newborns, were unexpectedly close to those obtained under general anesthesia (Table 5–3).

An intraocular pressure of 20 mm Hg or more by applanation in infants and children under anesthesia nearly always indicates pathology; the probability of such a pressure level being normal is less than 0.05 percent. Intraocular pressure in a healthy eye is variable, not fixed. The range of intraocular pressure variation in an individual eye is clinically much more important than the pressure at a given moment. The mean pressure of a normal infant eye is approximately 11 mm Hg (10–12 mm Hg) measured with the Draeger or Perkins applanation tonometer under general anesthesia. It must be emphasized that the individual's normal pressure (normative value) is of greater prognostic significance than is the statistical normal value. For example, an infant with a normative value of 9 mm Hg on healthy days may show a statistically normal pressure of 18 mm Hg at some later time. This increase of 9 mm Hg might be damaging to the optic nerve. At present we have no reliable means to estimate or to know the normative value of an eye in a given infant.

Many glaucoma cases in children under the age of 7 years are missed because of the unreliability of pressure testing in this age group. One should realize that an increase in optic disk cupping is easy to recognize early by ophthalmoscopy. Ophthalmoscopy is the most important procedure in the

Table 5–3

Intraocular Pressure by Applanation Tonometry in Infants and Young Children under General Anesthesia

Authors	Average of Normal (mm Hg)	Upper Limit of Normal (mm Hg)	Pathologic (mm Hg)
Weekers et al.[9]	10.23 ± 1.86	15–16	16
Dominguez et al.[10]	9.56 ± 2.66	17	20
Lee[11]	10.59 ± 1.94	15	18

diagnosis of glaucoma in children and in the assessment of the effectiveness of treatment. Cupping of the optic disk is produced in infants and children far earlier than it is in the adult at a comparable level of intraocular pressure. Often there will be severe cupping or damage of the optic disk at birth. The evidence of this early change is supported by the recent works of Shaffer, Weiss, Hetherington, and Richardson.[1-13-15] They stated that a cup/disk (c/d) ratio larger than 0.3 occurs in only 3.6 percent of normal infants and in 68 percent of infants with congenital glaucoma. They also reported that the prevalence of asymmetric c/d ratios was 2.3 perent in normal infants and 88 percent in infants with monocular congenital glaucoma. Our data fully support their statements. It is now clear that an asymmetric optic cup and a c/d ratio greater than 0.3 are found in less than 5 percent of normal infants and children. In addition, it is generally agreed that the cupping of the disk is of great value in evaluating the treatment and management of congenital glaucoma, especially infantile glaucoma.

Elevated intraocular pressure in infants and young children can produce damage to the optic disk in weeks or months, whereas damage to the disk in an adult takes place over a number of years at a comparable pressure level. Intermittent glaucomatous cupping associated with fluctuating intraocular pressure in infantile glaucoma is unlikely to be observable because of its transitory nature.

If the intraocular pressure is reduced to a normal level, an amazing reduction in the size of the optic disk cup can occur. But if intraocular pressure is not reduced, the cupping continues to progress; then damage and visual field loss begin, as in adults (Fig. 5–3). At this stage, normalization of pressure may bring reduction in cupping and field loss, but not complete recovery. The damage to visual function is permanent (Fig. 5–4).

Clinically, much attention has been directed toward the ocular signs and management of infants and children with congenital glaucoma, but the total care of the patient has been neglected. In addition to the classic ocular signs of congenital glaucoma, infants and children with glaucoma may occasionally present another important but unrecognized and unappreciated feature, pseudo mental retardation (PMR) or abnormal psychic behavior. It is because of these physical and psychic disturbances that some congenital glaucoma has been missed. What is worse, some of these children have been treated as retarded until useful vision has been lost. The psychic disturbances, such as abnormal psychophysical behavior and self-destructiveness, are really expressions of suffering from glaucoma, and they demand immediate attention from the mother as well as the physician. These psychophysical disturbances will either improve dramatically or disappear completely once the glaucoma is under control (Fig. 5–5).

Clinical symptoms of PMR syndrome are headaches, fullness of the

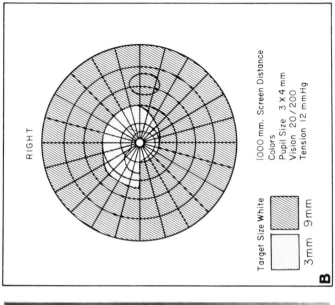

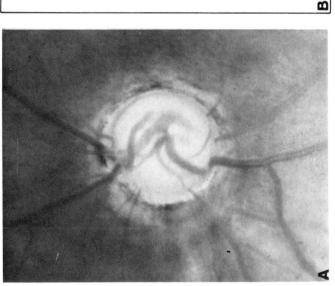

Figure 5–3. This 14-year-old boy with monocular congenital glaucoma received his first goniotomy at 3 years of age. Repeated surgical measures, as well as medical treatment, failed to control glaucoma. Trabeculotomy was performed at age 10 years, and glaucoma has since been stabilized. A: Optic disk is subtotally cupped and atrophic. B: Severe visual field loss remained unchanged after successful operation. There was no improvement in optic disk or visual function despite anatomically successful surgery. Visual acuity was 20/200, and intraocular pressure was 11 mm Hg by applanation without medication 4 years after operation.

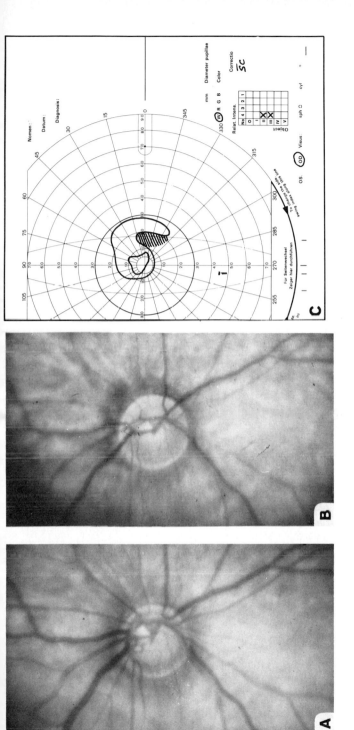

Figure 5–4. Photograph of optic disk in 11-year-old boy with far-advanced stage of aphakic glaucoma secondary to injury. There was an amazing reduction in the size of the optic disk 3 days after successful trabeculotomy surgery. However, visual function remained permanently damaged, despite successful arrest of the glaucoma. A and B: Optic disk and size of cupping, prior to operation (A shows marked cupped disk, C/d ratio = 0.8 × 0.9) and after operation (B shows normal disk appearance, c/d ratio = 0.3 × 0.4). C: Perimetry showed no improvement in visual field after the operation. Visual fields were identical before and 6 months after successful operation.

79

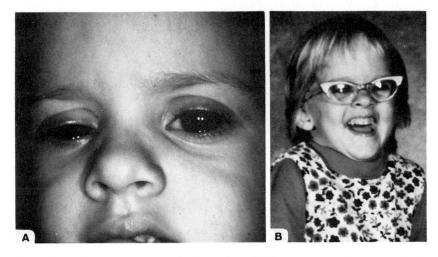

Figure 5–5.   Facial expression of patient with infantile glaucoma before (A) and after (B) successful operation. She demonstrated an unexpectedly dramatic personality reversal after operation. Her "retardation" symptoms had been related to or induced by increased intraocular pressure.

globe, reading difficulties, abnormal psychophysical behavior, "dullness," slow development in speech, and head nodding in children. The magnitude of PMR in children varies greatly, from a mild degree of psychic disturbance (crying baby, etc.) to a severe degree of self-abuse. Therefore parents, pediatrician, and ophthalmologist must be fully alert to the existence of psychic problems in children with congenital glaucoma. This is essential not only for preservation of vision but also for the child's well-being.

In addition, congenital glaucoma can present many problems to the child and family because of its uncertain prognosis, the threat of blindness, the necessarily prolonged contact with surgical procedures and treatment, and the requirement of a lifetime of follow-up examinations.

Diagnosis

Early detection and treatment are essential and most valuable in the successful management of congenital glaucoma, especially in the newborn infants under the age of 1 year. By early use of the newer surgical procedures and recent knowledge about congenital glaucoma and amblyopia, one can control the intraocular pressure and halt further deterioration in visual functions in at least 80 percent of cases. Useful vision may be preserved if the disease is recognized early and appropriate treatment is initiated. Early detection of congenital glaucoma that develops after the age of 1 year can be as difficult as the diagnosis of early adult glaucoma. Therefore the pediatrician, the primary care physician, and the ophthalmologist must be familiar with the early signs and symptoms of congenital glaucoma and must consistently be alert to its possibility, even though the disease is uncommon in any individual practice. Infantile glaucoma should be suspected and ruled out when tearing and photophobia are present. These symptoms usually result from early corneal edema and accompany corneal irritation secondary to elevated intraocular pressure.

The diagnosis of congenital glaucoma can be firmly established by evidence of elevated intraocular pressure, corneal edema, ruptures of Descemet's membrane, enlarged physiologic cupping of the optic disk, and buphthalmos. The presence of PMR symptoms is very helpful in detection of infantile glaucoma. Tonography, a method for estimating the trabecular patency in the human eye, is of less value and is difficult to perform in children. Visual field testing is not possible in younger children, but it is helpful and necessary in older children with juvenile glaucoma. Gonioscopy, a method for estimating the width, appearance, and anatomic configuration of the anterior chamber angle, should be done preoperatively in all cases. It is of great value in the differential diagnosis and in excluding the possibility of associated anomalies such as the anterior chamber cleavage syndrome of Reese, Axenfeld's syndrome, and others. In most infants the anterior chamber angle is open, and the apex of the angle is poorly developed. In monocular infantile glaucoma the angles of the eyes may seem identical. If the affected eye is buphthalmic, a rather characteristic segmentation or palisading of the pigment stroma at the periphery of the iris is present.

Other conditions that may involve congenital abnormalities of the filtration angle and congenital glaucoma follow, but they are discussed in more detail in other chapters: late congenital or infantile glaucoma; aniridia; Sturge-Weber syndrome; neurofibromatosis; Marfan's syndrome; Rieger's anomaly; Peter's anomaly; Lowe's syndrome; Pierre Robin syndrome; rubella syndrome.

Other conditions have congenitally normal filtration angle, but may have congenital glaucoma: persistent hyperplastic primary vitreous, unilateral (90 percent), associated with microphthalmia, vascularized mass behind the lens, visible ciliary processes, breaks in the posterior lens capsule, progressive posterior subcapsular cataract, shallowing of the anterior chamber, and vascularization of the iris; microcornea; retinoblastoma; retrolental fibroplasia; homocystinuria; spherophakia; juvenile xanthogranuloma; oculodental digital syndrome (trisomy 13); trisomy 18; mongolism (Down's syndrome); uveitis and keratitis; trauma (including recession of the chamber angle and hyphema, also postcataract obstruction); steroid-induced glaucoma.

In differential diagnosis there are many conditions that mimic congenital

Table 5–4
Signs of Primary Buphthalmos in Congenital Glaucoma

1. Elevated tension
2. Corneal size increases
3. Photophobia
4. Corneal opacities (stromal edema, ruptures in Descemet's membrane)
5. Cornea flattened; astigmatism against the rule
6. Angle dysgenesis (mesodermal tissue obscures angle structures)
7. c/d ratio may exceed 0.4
8. Bilateral in about two-thirds of cases, but asymmetric
9. May be autosomal recessive (60% males)
10. Familial occurrence unusual
11. Visual prognosis poor
12. PMR and psychic disturbances

glaucomas and that must always be excluded. The most common conditions are megalocornea (Tables 5–4 and 5–5), high or excessive myopia, congenital idiopathic corneal edema, rubella, syphilitic keratitis, birth injuries of the cornea, mucopolysaccharidoses, connective tissue diseases, and phakomatoses. Therefore a careful eye examination under general anesthesia is essential; it usually establishes the diagnosis.

Briefly, the cause of congenital glaucoma must be differentiated from the following causes: inflammation; systemic diseases; trauma; skin disease; corneal dystrophy; genetic disorders; birth injuries; medication.

Corneal diameter and disk cupping often reflect the level of intraocular pressure. The method of comparative ophthalmoscopy is of great importance in establishing the diagnosis and in evaluating the functional status of infantile glaucoma patients, who are prone to follow a more asymmetric course than

Table 5–5
Clinical Features of Physiologic Large Cornea (Megalocornea)

1. Normal tension
2. Corneal size constant
3. Asymptomatic
4. Central cornea clear
5. Corneal curve normal or increased; astigmatism with the rule
6. Angle normal; may contain iris processes
7. c/d ratio less than 0.4
8. Bilateral and symmetric
9. Sex-linked recessive (92% male)
10. Familial occurrence common
11. Visual prognosis good
12. Mental and psychic condition normal

adults with glaucoma. An optic disk having physiologic cupping with a diameter at least one-half to two-thirds that of the disk occurs infrequently and should be considered as pathologic until proven otherwise. This is especially true in the presence of asymmetric optic disk cupping.

Buphthalmos in infantile glaucoma usually presents a number of signs *(vide supra)* that are valuable in distinguishing primary buphthalmos and congenital glaucoma (Table 5–4) from secondary buphthalmos and associated ocular pathology (Table 5–5).

Enlargement of the cornea induced by glaucoma in infants must be differentiated from the benign form of congenitally large cornea (megalocornea). The signs and clinical features of megalocornea listed in Table 5–5 are helpful in the differential diagnosis. Secondary glaucoma related to dislocation of the lens and the phakomatoses are discussed in other chapters.

Corneal haze in newborn infants requires total pediatric evaluation. Causes of corneal haze in infants and children can be related to any one of the following:

1.   Mucopolysaccharidoses (Hurler, Scheie, Morquio, Maroteaux-Lamy, and β-Glucuronidase deficiency)
2.   Cystinosis
3.   Hereditary corneal dystrophy
4.   Interstitial keratitis
5.   Rubella syndrome
6.   Congenital glaucoma
7.   Birth injury, trauma
8.   Intraocular mass lesion or hemorrhage
9.   Anterior segment malformation
10.   Trisomy 13
11.   Inborn errors of metabolism
12.   Stromal dystrophy
13.   Medication (topical steroids, etc.)

The conditions to be differentiated from congenital glaucoma are the following: megalocornea (Table 5–5); forceps injury; keratitis; mucopolysaccharidosis; cystinosis; congenital hereditary corneal dystrophy; hereditary connective tissue disorders.

OCULAR INJURIES

Glaucoma secondary to ocular trauma is a fairly common occurrence in children. The most common causes of secondary glaucoma related to ocular injuries are hyphema, anterior uveitis associated with dislocated lens, iridodialysis, and chamber angle recession associated with tears in the trabecular meshwork. Several ocular complications may occur: retinal detachment, vitreous hemorrhage and/or vitreous traction, severe glaucoma and hematogenous pigmentation to the cornea, iris and corneal adhesion, and seclusion of the pupil. Secondary hemorrhage or rebleeding is usually worse than primary hyphema. Prompt and appropriate management is essential in reducing the incidence of severe ocular complication and ensuring better visual prognosis. Visual results depend on the following factors:

1. Corneal scratching, hematogenous pigmentation
2. Glaucoma, peripheral anterior synechiae, recessing of the angle, degenerated red blood cells (erythroclastic), and inflammatory reaction of the trabecular tissues
3. Inflammatory pupillary membrane
4. Traumatic cataract, contusion, or perforating injury
5. Vitreous hemorrhage and/or vitreous traction
6. Retinal damage:
   A. Macular edema, cystodegeneration, commotio retinae
   B. Retinal detachment
   C. Choroidal rupture
7. Optic nerve damage:
   A. Papilledema
   B. Traumatic optic neuritis, and/or
   C. Ischemic optic neuropathy

TREATMENT

The aim of treatment for any form of glaucoma is to prevent loss of visual function. The only effective form of treatment for congenital glaucoma is surgery. Goniotomy, a traditional procedure performed under direct visualization, is the safest and most effective treatment presently available for control of infantile glaucoma. The technique is relatively simple and rapid, and it may be repeated at least four times with little damage to the integrity of the eye. If goniotomy fails, the intact external eye remains suitable for other procedures, such as external trabeculotomy or a filtering operation.

In goniotomy, an incision is made within the anterior aspect of the chamber angle meshwork, which makes Schlemm's canal accessible to the aqueous humor and lowers the intraocular pressure.[16] Usually, more than one goniotomy is necessary. Once pressure is lowered to normal, the prognosis for glaucoma control and visual function is good. If repeated goniotomies fail to control glaucoma, trabeculotomy is indicated. In trabeculotomy a trabeculotome is introduced into Schlemm's canal and swung into the anterior chamber, producing an opening between Schlemm's canal and the anterior chamber.

Surgery should be prompt. Long-term medical treatment is of little value, for it only permits the eye to deteriorate because of poor response to medical therapy in infantile glaucoma. However, short-term medical therapy is beneficial between surgeries. Surgery will control intraocular pressure in 80–85 percent of uncomplicated cases, and where goniotomy and/or goniopuncture or trabeculotomy fail, a filtering procedure or cyclocryotherapy can be used.

It should also be emphasized here that infantile glaucoma can exist at birth and that when it is arrested it nearly always results in myopia. Amblyopia will soon develop in the majority of these eyes if appropriate management is not instituted in time. The management of amblyopia has been described in another chapter. The treatment of amblyopia should be integrated with surgical measures in the management of congenital glaucoma.

Medical therapy with Phospholine Iodide or Humorsol should be stopped 2 weeks prior to any anesthesia because serum butyrocholinesterase is depressed in these patients. It is well known that succinylcholine depends on butyrocholinesterase to hydrolyze it to succinate and acetate ions and thereby terminate its activity. Prolonged apnea may result if succinylcholine is given to a patient still under anticholinesterase medication.

A complete preoperative pediatric evaluation is necessary to rule out possible systemic disease, including cardiac status, metabolic inborn errors, and rubella infections. It has been recognized that there is a high correlation of eye and systemic involvement in these conditions.

Medical Therapy

The dosage of antiglaucoma agents used in infants and children should not be calculated by the child's age because of weight variations in children of the same age; dosage should be determined according to either weight or surface area of the child. In general, either Clark's weight formula or Augsberger's rule by weight is preferred. Clark's formula by weight is widely used for children 2 years of age or older:

$$\text{pediatric dose} = \frac{\text{child's weight (kg or lb)} \times \text{adult dose}}{(70 \text{ kg or } 150 \text{ lb})}$$

Augsberger's rule by weight is useful for children under 2 years of age:

$$\text{pediatric dose} = \text{child's weight in kg} \times 1.5 + 10$$

Example: A child weighing 5 kg would receive $\times$ 1.5 $\times$ 10 = 17.5 percent of the adult dose.

The side effects of common drugs used in the treatment of glaucoma are many and cannot be covered adequately in this volume. In order to become familiar with the side effects of such medications, one needs a pharmacology review.[5] The most common drug-related complications are miotic-induced accommodation spasm, cataract; and systemic adverse effects induced by carbonic anhydrase inhibitors, such as paresthesias, gastrointestinal upsets, malaise, and loss of physical initiative. However, in children, miotic-induced pseudo iris cysts are more common, and occurrences of posterior synechiae of the iris and/or transient lens opacities are much less frequent. With osmotic agents, anginalike chest pain and allergic reactions may occur with mannitol infusion; hyperglycemia (or glycosuria) and convulsive seizure with disorientation may be seen with oral glycerol administration.

For convenience, the drugs commonly used in the management of congenital glaucoma patients will be described briefly, even though this is basically a surgical disease. Drugs to dilate the pupil and sedatives for the eye examination will also be described in this chapter.

MIOTICS

Cholinergic drugs (parasympathomimetics) act directly on the nerve endings; they are short-acting agents. Commonly used miotics are pilocarpine and carbachol:

1. Pilocarpine hydrochloride (0.5 percent to 4 percent); 1 percent and 2 percent are common as drops, q. 4–6 hr
2. Carbachol (0.75 percent, 1.5 percent, and 3 percent) drops q. 4–8 hr

Anticholinesterase drugs inhibit the enzyme cholinesterase; they may be short-acting (eserine) or long-acting (echothiopate and Humorsol). They have more side effects than cholinergic agents.

1. Physostigmine (eserine) 0.25, 0.50, 0.75, and 1 percent aqueous solution, 0.5 percent oil solution, 0.25 percent ointment
2. Echothiopate iodide (Phospholine Iodide) 0.03 percent, 0.06 percent, 0.125 percent, 0.25 percent drops q. 12–24
3. Demecarium bromide (Humorsol) 0.125 percent, 0.25 percent solution, drops q. 12–24 hr

MYDRIATICS

Adrenergic drugs (sympathomimetics) lower intraocular pressure by decreasing aqueous formation and in some instances by increasing outflow facility.

1. l-Epinephrine, topical, 1 drop q. 12–24 hr

    a.   Hydrochloride (Glaucon 1 or 2 percent, Epifrin 0.25 percent, 0.5 percent, 1 percent, 2 percent)

    b.   Borate (Eppy or Epinal) 0.5 or 1 percent

    c.   Bitartrate (Epitrate) 1 or 2 percent

2.   Phenylephrine hydrochloride (Neo-Synephrine) 2.5 percent and 10 percent is used to dilate pupils for fundus and ocular media examination. It has less effect on aqueous formation than does epinephrine; it is seldom used for treatment of glaucoma. However, it has been used as an adjunct to miotic agents.

CARBONIC ANHYDRASE INHIBITORS

The following four agents are often used in the management of congenital glaucoma. These agents reduce intraocular pressure by decreasing the rate of aqueous formation.

1.   Diamox is the most commonly used carbonic anhydrase inhibitor because it has been studied and used over many years.

    a.   Newborns: up to 15 mg/kg (2.25 lb) of body weight in divided doses

    b.   Infants under 1 year: 5–10 mg/kg body weight q. 6 hr

    c.   Children 2 years and up: 10–30 mg/kg body weight q. 1 hr (about one-fifth adult dose)

2.   Daranide: 2–8 mg/kg/24 hr orally in 3–4 divided doses

3.   Cardarase: 4–15 mg/kg/24 hr orally in 3–4 divided doses

4.   Neptazane: 2–8 mg/kg/24 hr orally in 2–3 divided doses

Potassium replacement in infants and children is usually not necessary because of the potassium contained in the daily milk intake and in baby food and because of the short term application of these agents. Occasionally potassium replacement may be necessary, in which case Kaon elixir (teaspoonful q. 12–24 hr) may be prescribed.

OSMOTIC AGENTS

It has been generally accepted that a rapid increase in plasma osmolarity will extract fluid from the eye and shrink the vitreous, resulting in a reduction in intraocular volume and pressure that will last for 3–4 hr. The commonly used osmotics are glycerol and mannitol.

Osmotic agents seldom are indicated in newborns or infants with congenital glaucoma secondary to ocular injuries and postoperative complications.

1.   Glycerol (glycerine) 50 percent.

    a.   Young children: 0.75–1 mg/kg oral; the sickeningly sweet taste of glycerol can be masked by mixing the 50 percent diluent with cracked ice and lemon or orange juice

    b.   Older children: 1.0–1.5 mg/kg

2. Mannitol 20 percent IV
    a. Infants: use 10 percent 0.5–1.5 g/kg IV at rate of 5 cc/min or 60 drops/min
    b. Older children: 20 percent solution can be used (same dosage as above)

AGENTS FOR EYE EXAMINATION AND DILATING
THE PUPIL

1. Newborns
    a. Tropicamide (Mydriacyl) 0.5 percent
    b. Cyclopentolate (Cyclogyl) 0.5 percent
    c. Phenylephrine HCl (Neo-Synephrine) 2.5 percent
2. Infants
    a. Mydriacyl 0.5 percent
    b. Cyclogyl 0.5 percent
    c. Neo-Synephrine 2.5 percent
3. Older children
    a. Mydriacyl 0.5–1.0 percent
    b. Cyclogyl 0.5–1.0 percent
    c. Neo-Synephrine 2.5–5 percent

In general, it is advisable not to use more than 4 drops (or more than 2 drops in each eye) for pupillary dilation in order to avoid adverse drug reaction and toxicity.

SEDATION

A sedation mixture may be used for ophthalmic diagnosis and therapy in uncooperative and/or selected young children. Each 1 cc of the sedative mixture contains the following: meperidine (Demerol) 25 mg (made from ½ cc of 50 mg/ml ampule); chlorpromazine (Thorazine) 6.25 mg (made from ¼ cc of 25 mg/ml ampule); promethazine (Phenergan) 6.25 mg (made from ¼ cc of 25 mg/ml ampule). The dosage schedule is as follows:

Body Weight (lb)	Dose of Sedative Mixture (cc)
15	0.5
20	0.75
25	0.85
30	1.0
40	1.5
50	1.6
60	1.7
70	1.8
80	1.9
90	2.0

PROGNOSIS

In any form of glaucoma the prognosis is improved by prompt diagnosis and normalization of intraocular pressure. This is particularly true in infantile and juvenile glaucomas. Delay in treatment results in rapid enlargement of the cornea, with breaks or tears in Descemet's membrane that can produce scarring in the visual axis and irregular astigmatism. The optic disk is rapidly cupped and destroyed if elevated ocular pressure persists.

The prognosis for a good visual result is best when the disease develops in infants from 3 to 6 months of age who at the time of surgery show little ocular enlargement or optic nerve damage. Early diagnosis and prompt surgery are therefore of foremost importance.

Continuing care. When intraocular pressure has been normalized, there is no further enlargement of the corneal diameter and optic disk cup. Such a case is considered to be arrested. No case of glaucoma should be considered as permanently cured. There will be occasional elevation of pressure in eyes years after a seemingly successful surgery. It is of vital impor tance to continue to examine these patients every year or every 2 years of life.

MALIGNANT HYPERTHERMIA ASSOCIATED WITH OPHTHALMIC SURGERY

When an infant is scheduled for an eye examination under anesthesia and surgery, the possibilities for developing malignant hyperthermia during the surgery should be considered. Malignant hyperthermia is one of the most catastrophic complications that can develop during normal and well-conducted administration of surgical anesthesia. It is a rare and often lethal surgical complication. The mortality rate is high, and the body temperature control mechanism in an infant under the age of 3 months has yet to be developed. Therefore the danger must always be kept in mind, and it must be explained to the parents as part of the surgical risk involved.[17-23] The important points relevant to malignant hyperthermia are as follows:

1. It is characterized by high fever (108°F to 114°F), usually with skeletal muscle rigidity during general anesthesia. The usual symptoms are sudden tachycardia, tachypnea, and massive respiratory and metabolic acidosis far exceeding the ability of the lungs to clear through normal pathways.
2. Treatment involves reduction of the elevated temperature, as well as correction of the physiological abnormality associated with the hyperthermia episode; intravenous cooling, administration of sodium bicarbonate, and drug therapy may be required.

3. The mechanism of this syndrome is probably due to inhibition of calcium transport in muscle, which leads to hypercalcemia and hyperthermia. There is no reliable means to predict its occurrence clinically, but genetic factors, preexisting congenital muscular defects, and latent myopathy predispose the patient to malignant hyperthermia. A familial history of unexplained death during surgery is suggestive.
4. Malignant hyperthermia occurs in 1 of 14,000 cases, and the death rate is 65–70 percent.
5. Occurrence is related to the use of potent inhalation agents and skeletal muscle relaxants.
6. It can be expected in surgery for strabismus or blepharoptosis as well as congenital cataract, congenital glaucoma, and even a routine eye examination where general anesthesia is used.

Management
1. Reduce elevated temperature
   a. External cooling: immersion in ice and water; saltwater towels; electric fans
   b. Internal cooling: intravenous refrigerated Ringer's lactate; irrigation of peritoneal cavity with refrigerated Ringer's lactate
   c. Increase body heat loss: convert anesthetic system to nonrebreathing
2. Prevent shivering by use of small intravenous doses of chlorpromazine hydrochloride or meperidine
3. Correct physiologic abnormalities associated with the hyperthermia
   a. Metabolic acidosis: correct base defect
   b. Respiratory acidosis: hyperventilation
   c. Hypoxemia: ventilate with high oxygen concentration
   d. Reduce myoplasmic calcium: infuse procaine amide
   e. Counteract hypovolemia and support cardiovascular system: infuse Ringer's lactate

JUVENILE GLAUCOMA

Juvenile glaucoma is a distinct clinical entity because it occurs between the ages of 6 and 30 years, and about 40 percent of cases occur between the ages of 16 and 20 years; 50–80 percent of such patients are myopic. It occurs more often in males, and there is no enlargement of the eye or buphthalmos.

Incidence

No recent survey has been reported. The incidence of juvenile glaucoma is about 0.01 percent at Wills Eye Hospital. A strong family history of open-angle glaucoma has been reported.

Symptoms

Juvenile glaucoma has no specific symptoms; it often runs the insidious course of adult open-angle glaucoma. A common presenting symptom is poor vision at school; thus there may be referral by a school nurse for eye examination. Occasional dull headache, fullness of the eyeball, and inability to withstand long hours of reading or close-up work have been observed. More often the glaucoma is discovered accidentally, and then only after marked glaucomatous optic disk cupping and severe visual field loss have occurred. Externally, the corneal diameter is normal; it may even be smaller than normal. There is no buphthalmos, tearing, or photophobia. There is no obvious external ocular pathology.

Diagnosis

Early diagnosis is essential because present-day treatment, if employed early, can control the intraocular pressure and arrest the disease in the major ity of cases. In the absence of obvious ocular pathology, the presence of elevated intraocular pressure, enlargement of the optic cup, and visual field changes are important diagnostically in the detection of juvenile glaucoma.

Intraocular Pressure

The degree of elevation of intraocular pressure is moderate to high, usually in the range of 30–40 mm Hg. Characteristically, intraocular pressure in the juvenile form of glaucoma tends to fluctuate, with greater day-to-day variations. Rapid rises in pressure, accompanied by halos (rainbowlike), may occur more frequently in juvenile glaucoma than in adult open-angle glaucoma in older individuals. Intermittent pressure elevation has been reported. Tonography usually indicates impairment in the outflow facility of aqueous humor. Blurring of vision, with or without halos, occurs when the corneal epithelial edema that is secondary to increased pressure develops.

Optic Disk and Visual Field

In general, glaucomatous cupping of the disk is more severe in the juvenile age group than in adult or older persons. Usually the pressure elevation is long-standing, and thus marked cupping and atrophy are common.

The glaucomatous cupping in the juvenile age group may be atypical, especially in the presence of myopia. The disk cup, because of anatomic differentiation at the tissue level of lamina cribrosa, tends to be shallow and broad and therefore difficult to detect. Children with rapid progressive myopia should be susepcted of having glaucoma unless proven otherwise.

Visual field defects usually are related to the status of the optic disk and they occur at advanced stages of glaucoma. Arcuate scotoma or papillomacular nerve fiber bundle defects are rarely seen without advanced cupping, although a surprising amount of central cupping may occur at times with no demonstrable visual field defect unless the cupping is extended to the disk margin. Early field defects are detectable in the central 30° area. Any child with a suspiciously cupped optic disk (unusually large or asymmetric with c/d ratio greater than one-half of the horizontal disk diameter) should have a visual field examination, particularly when the child is cooperative and is old enough for a reliable field test.

The optic disk damage and field defect may progress, as does impairment of vision, unless a desirable or acceptable level of intraocular pressure is achieved medically or surgically. Central vision, however, is retained until the glaucoma is far advanced. Therefore children or young adults are frequently unaware of visual loss until they are practically blind. In the presence of typical glaucomatous visual field defects (arcuate, Bjerrum, or paracentral scotoma) without optic disk cupping, conditions such as pituitary tumors, tabes dorsalis, optic disk pit and colobomas of the choroid and retina adjacent to the optic disk should be considered.

Treatment

Juvenile glaucoma is more difficult to treat successfully than other types of glaucoma. Response to medical therapy is invariably poor, and surgery is usually necessary. In cases that seemingly do well with the medical approach, lifetime preservation of usual vision can hardly be expected. Undesirable side effects of miotics and other agents tend to make patients less faithful in taking their medication; hence there are more failures. However, medical therapy can be used effectively initially and between surgeries, especially in cases with a favorable response to the medication. Newer compounds and newer drug delivery systems can also be used selectively in the management of juvenile glaucoma.

Indications for surgery are basically similar to those in adult open-angle glaucoma with progressive optic disk cupping and loss of visual field. However, early surgery in children with poorly controlled intraocular pressure and disk damage should be performed because of their long life expectancy; also, the optic disk is less tolerant to high pressure than an adult disk under comparable conditions.

Surgical Procedures

Cases with early onset do better with goniotomy; late-onset cases do better with trabeculotomy or trabeculectomy. In general, goniotomy, followed by trabeculotomy, is best; results following trabeculectomy have been disappointing. Cyclocryotherapy can be used in selected cases or when other conventional surgical measures fail. Laser trabeculotomy has produced only transitory pressure reduction in less than one-third of reported cases and it is not widely used.

Prognosis and Follow-up

All juvenile glaucoma patients require indefinite periods of follow-up and should be treated as infantile glaucoma patients until the age of 30 years. It is not unusual to see a child lose total visual function due to recurrence of glaucoma a few years after apparently successful surgery. Periodic optic disk and visual field examinations are essential and are most helpful. Intraocular pressure may vary at times, and there may be difficulties in obtaining reliable readings in children.

REFERENCES

1. Shaffer RN, Weiss DL: Congenital and Pediatric Glaucomas. St Louis, CV Mosby, 1970
2. Kwitko ML: Glaucoma in Infants and Children. New York, Appleton-Century-Crofts, 1973
3. Chandler PA, Grant WM: Lectures on Glaucoma. Philadelphia, Lea & Febiger, 1965
4. Kolker AE, Hetherington J Jr: Becker and Shaffer's Diagnosis and Therapy of Glaucoma (ed 4). St Louis CV Mosby, 1976
5. Havener WH: Ocular Pharmacology (ed 3). St Louis, CV Mosby 1974
6. Anderson J: Hydrophthalmia or Congenital Glaucoma: Its Causes, Treatment and Cure. London, Cambridge University press, 1939
7. Lehrfeld L, Reber J: Glaucoma at the Wills Hospital, 1926–1936. Arch Ophthalmol 18:712, 1937
8. Lamb HD: Hydrophthalmus. Am J Ophthalmol 8:784, 1925
9. Weekers R, Prijot E, Henrotte J, Engels G: Ocular pressure of young children during anesthesia. Arch Ophthalmol (Paris) 34:241–250, 1974
10. Dominguez A, Banos MS, Alvarez MG, Contra GF, Quintela FB: Intraocular pressure measurement in infants under general anesthesia. Am J Ophthalmol 78:110–116, 1974
11. Lee PF: Unpublished data, 1976
12. Radtke ND, Cohan BE: Intraocular pressure measurement in the newborn.Am J Ophthalmol 78:501–504, 1974
13. Richardson KT, Shaffer RN: Optic nerve cupping in congenital glaucoma. Am J Ophthalmol 62:507–509, 1966
14. Richardson KT: Optic nerve symmetry in normal newborn infants. Invest Ophthalmol 7:137–140, 1968

15. Shaffer RN, Hetherington J Jr: The glaucomatous disc in infants. Trans Am Acad Ophthalmol Otolaryingol 73:929–935, 1969

16. Barkan O: Technic of goniotomy for congenital glaucoma. Trans Am Acad Ophthalmol 52:210, 1948

17. Beasley H: Hyperthermia associated with ophthalmic surgery. Am J Ophthalmol 77:76–79, 1974

18. Snow J: Malignant hyperthermia during anesthesia and surgery. Arch Ophthalmol 85:407, 1970

19. Rowell RR: Malignant hyperthermia. Arch Ophthalmol 85:638, 1971

20. Aldrete JA, Padfield A, Solomon CC, Rubright MW: Possible predictive tests for malignant hyperthermia during anesthesia. JAMA 215:1465, 1971

21. Wang JK, Moffit EA; Rosevear JW: Oxidative phosphorylation in acute hyperthermia. Anesthesiology: 30:439, 1969

22. Britt BA, Kalow W: Malignant hyperthermia. A statistical review. Can Anaesth Soc J 17:293, 1970

23. Ryan J: Physicians tend to miss malignant hyperthermia. JAMA 235:238, 1976

John F. Griffin, M.D.

6
Pediatric Neuro-ophthalmology

VISUAL FIELDS

The normal monocular field extends laterally 100 degrees, downward 75 degrees, and medially and upward 60 degrees. Isopters are contour lines of geodetic plots of this visual field; they are quite constant in size and shape for a particular-size target. Large bright targets are used to examine the outer limits of the visual field, whereas the central area is best explored with smaller and dimmer targets.

For infants and young children, in whom sophisticated testing is not possible, useful clinical information can be gained by visual field testing appropriate to the age of the child. A child who has the same degree of vision in each eye will not object to occlusion of either eye; if vision is reduced in one eye from any cause, the child will vigorously resent covering the sound eye. Infants over 3 months of age with intact vision will make visually elicited head and eye movements in the direction of a small light or brightly colored toy presented silently in each quadrant of the visual field. This fixation reflex provides a mechanism for testing gross visual function in the peripheral field.

Determination of confrontation fields is extremely valuable in older children. The patient sits or stands an arm's length away from the examiner with the patient's eyes on the same level. The left eye is covered first, and the examiner's left eye is used as a fixation point. The patient's visual field is then compared with that of the examiner. The test object chosen will depend on the degree of visual acuity, as well as on the degrees of intelligence and cooperation; it can vary in size, e.g., the extended fingers of one hand, or a small white-headed hat pin. The target is moved from the blind area to the seeing area around the circumference of the patient's visual field. Hemianopic, quadrantic, and central defects can be surveyed accurately.

After the age of 5 years, intelligent children often are able to cooperate for more formal testing on the Goldmann perimeter or tangent screen.

Visual Field Defects in Retinal Lesions

If the lesion involves only the *rod-and-cone layer* of the retina, the visual field defect (Fig. 6–1) will correspond exactly to the retinal defect in position, shape, extent, and intensity. The retinal lesion, either inflammatory or degenerative, is usually visible with the ophthalmoscope.

When the *nerve fibers* of the retina are involved, the defect corresponds to the field represented by the fibers that are obstructed; this results in an arcuate or Bjerrum visual field defect (Fig. 6–2).

Visual Field Defects in Optic Nerve Lesions

With *central defects* the scotoma (Fig. 6–3) involves the central visual field. It may vary in size from 2 degrees to 40 degrees. The peripheral field is uninvolved, but in larger defects a breakthrough to the periphery from the central area may occur. The most common causes are inflammatory, demyelinating, toxic, or compressive lesions affecting the nerve.

A central defect that extends to involve the blind spot is called a *centrocecal defect* (Fig. 6–4). Centrocecal defects are seen in toxic affectations of the optic nerve, but they also may occur in inflammatory and demyelinating disease.

Nerve fiber bundle defects extend from the blind spot in an arcuate or scimitar-shaped fashion corresponding to the nerve fiber layer of the retina. This is the classic field defect of glaucoma (Fig. 6-2).

Altitudinal defects are caused by occlusion of one of the posterior ciliary arteries that supply the optic nerve. The upper or lower half of the visual field will be lost (Fig. 6-5), with a clear horizontal demarcation between the seeing and nonseeing areas. In childhood this is most commonly produced by blood dyscrasias.

An *enlarged blind spot* is caused by displacement of the retinal elements due to edema of the optic nerve head. It is seen in papilledema, but it also may be caused by drusen of the optic nerve head, myelinated nerve fibers, temporal crescents in myopia, glaucoma, and developmental defects of the optic nerve.

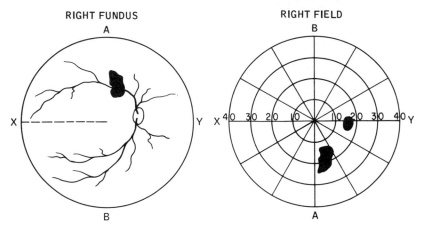

RIGHT FUNDUS
A

RIGHT FIELD
B

Figure 6-1.   The upper temporal retinal lesion produces a field defect which is seen by the patient as being below and slightly nasal to the blind spot.

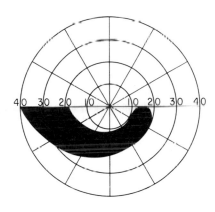

Figure 6-2.   The arcuate scotoma classically seen in glaucoma due to damage to the nerve fiber layer at the optic nerve head.

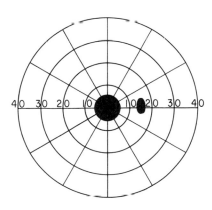

Figure 6-3.   Central scotoma most commonly seen in retrobulbar neuritis.

97

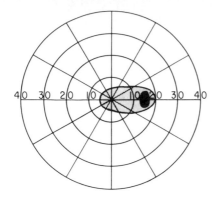

Figure 6-4. A centrocecal visual field defect charactersitic of toxic amblyopia. (From Harrington, David O.: The visual fields, ed. 4, St. Louis, 1976, The C. V. Mosby Co.)

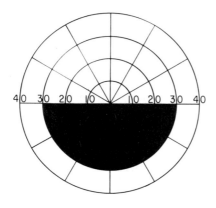

Figure 6-5. Inferior altitudinal visual field defect due to occlusion of one of the posterior ciliary arteries supplying the optic nerve. (From Harrington, David O.: The visual fields, ed. 4, St. Louis, 1976, The C. V. Mosby Co.

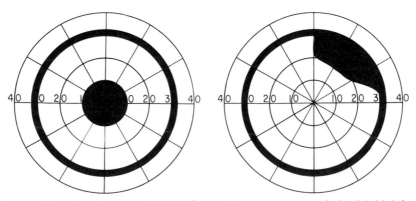

Figure 6-6. Central scotoma in the left eye with a upper temporal visual field defect in the right eye. This is due to compression of the left optic nerve where it enters the chiasm, with involvement of the lower nasal fibers (subserving the upper temporal field) from the right eye.

Visual Field Defects with Chiasmal Lesions

Lesions at the *anterior angle of the chiasm* may produce a central scotoma in the ipsilateral eye and an upper temporal defect in the contralateral eye due to involvement of the lower nasal fibers that loop forward in the contralateral optic nerve in the genu of Willebrand (Fig. 6–6).

Lesions involving the *body of the chiasm* produce bitemporal defects that may be peripheral or central (Fig. 6–8). Pressure from below (usually caused by a pituitary adenoma) causes an upper temporal defect, whereas pressure from above causes a lower temporal defect (Fig. 6-7A,B).

Lesions of the *posterior angle of the chiasm* where the macular fibers cross may cause a bitemporal hemianopic scotoma (Fig. 6–8).

Pressure on the *lateral aspect of the chiasm* will cause a binasal hemianopia (Fig. 6-9).

Visual Field Defects with Optic Tract Lesions

Postchiasmal lesions cause homonymous hemianopia (loss of vision in the two right halves or two left halves of the visual fields). The hemianopia due to a tract lesion is typically incongruous (not the same in each eye) (Fig. 6–10).

Visual Field Defects with Temporal Lobe Lesions

Lesions in the temporal lobe region produce incongruous wedge-shaped upper quadrantic homonymous defects, more easily remembered as "pie in the sky" (Fig. 6–11).

Visual Field Defects with Parietal Lobe Lesions

The homonymous field defect is usually denser below, and congruity is more marked (Fig. 6–12). Remember that in nondominant parietal lobe lesions a large tumor may produce subtle findings, and a visual field defect may not be noted unless simultaneous stimulation of the two half fields is done.

Visual Field Defects and Occipital Lobe Lesions

Homonymous defects, which are extremely congruous, occur without other evidence of neurologic or neuro-ophthalmic signs and symptoms (Fig. 6–13). Macular sparing in which the central area is intact for about 5 degrees frequently occurs.

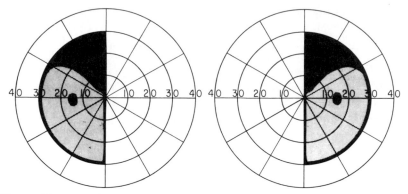

Figure 6-7A. A complete bitemporal visual field defect which is denser above, characteristic of compression of the chiasm from below, as is seen in a pituitary tumor.

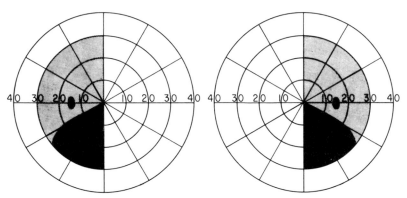

Figure 6-7B. Complete bitemporal visual field defect which is denser below due to compression of the chiasm from above.

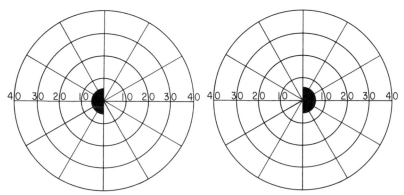

Figure 6-8. A bitemporal hemianopic scotoma seen in compression of the posterior angle of the chiasm where the macular fibers cross. (From Harrington, David O.: The visual fields, ed. 4, St. Louis, 1976, The C. V. Mosby Co.)

100

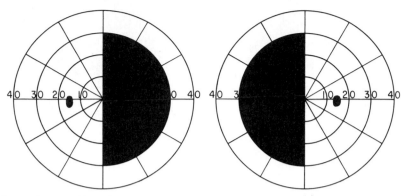

Figure 6-9. A binasal hemianopsia caused by compression of the uncrossed temporal fibers of both eyes.

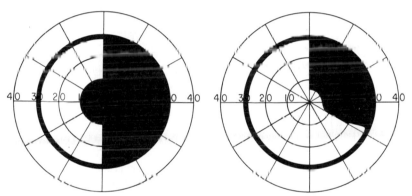

Figure 6-10. An incongruous homonymous hemianopsia with involvement of central vision in the left eye seen in a lesion of the optic tract.

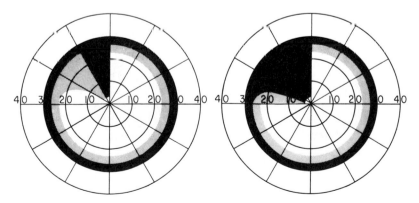

Figure 6-11. "Pie in the sky," which is due to a lesion in the right temporal lobe.

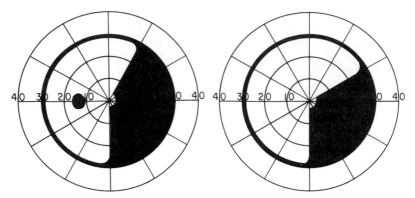

Figure 6-12. Congruity becomes more marked with a lesion closer to the occipital lobe. Here a left parietal lobe lesion has caused a right homonymous defect which is denser inferiorly. (From Harrington, David O.: The visual fields, ed. 4, St. Louis, 1976, The C. V. Mosby Co.)

Functional Visual Field Defects

Children over the age of 10 years may complain of decreased vision in one or both eyes. Needless investigations may be undertaken and much anxiety engendered if the functional nature of the visual loss is not recognized. The visual field defects do not resemble those found in organic lesions of the visual pathways. Functional visual field defects commonly resemble a contracting spiral or a star-shaped figure, or they may be contracted to less than 10 degrees for all sizes of targets and be the same at different distances from the target screen (Fig. 6–15).

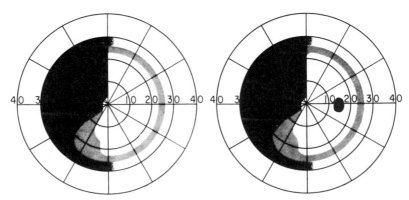

Figure 6-13. An absolutely congruous left homonymous visual field defect due to a lesion of the right occipital lobe. (From Harrington, David O.: The Visual fields, ed. 4, St. Louis, 1976, The C. V. Mosby Co.)

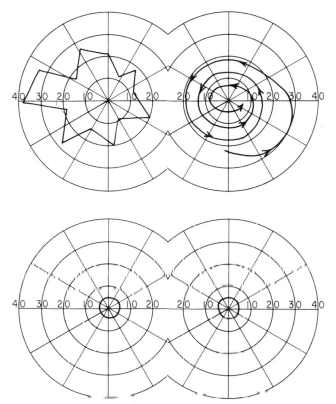

Figure 6-14.   The typical visual field defects seen in nonorganic
visual loss, contracting spiral, stellate, and marked contraction of
the visual field.

OPTIC NERVE

Anomalies of the optic nerve, either developmental in origin or associated with refractive errors, are frequent sources of confusion. In a moderately myopic patient the optic nerve may appear larger and slightly pale
temporally and thus may simulate optic atrophy. In moderate to severe degrees of hyperopia the optic nerve often appears elevated and hyperemic and
may be confused with papilledema.

Drusen

Drusen or hyaline bodies of the optic nerve are easily visible in adults as
discrete, highly refractile glowing masses on the optic nerve head. In children
they are frequently buried deep in the substance of the disk producing eleva-

tion of the optic nerve and blurring of the disk margins. Visual acuity is usually normal. Enlargement of the blind spot or defects in the inferonasal visual field are commonly seen on tangent screen testing. Drusen are inherited in an irregular dominant fashion; thus examination of other family members when a child has a suspiciously elevated optic nerve may reveal obvious drusen.

Medullated Nerve Fibers

Medullated nerve fibers appear as creamy white extensions of the normal optic nerve. The feathery edge and superficial location in the nerve fiber layer are characteristic and should serve to distinguish this condition from optic atrophy.

Hyaloid Vessels

Remnants of the hyaloid arterial system (Bergmeister's papilla) may persist on the disk and may be associated with hyperplastic glial remnants that may simulate papilledema.

Congenital Optic Nerve Head Tilting

Congenital tilting of the optic nerve head may produce a bitemporal visual field defect that has been mistaken for that caused by chiasmal compression. The optic nerve itself is tilted at a 45-degree angle, and the vessels exit from the disk in an abnormal fashion. The visual field defect does not respect the vertical midline as in true chiasmal compression, but instead is limited to the smallest targets and slopes across the vertical meridian in an irregular fashion.

Hypoplastic Optic Nerves

Hypoplasia of the optic nerves may be bilateral or unilateral, and visual acuity may be normal or severely reduced. If visual acuity is normal, minimally hypoplastic nerves may be unrecognized. The more extreme examples are about one-third the size of a normal optic nerve; they have a grayish appearance and frequently are surrounded by a pigmented halo. If there is no associated neurologic deficit, further studies are not indicated. Optic nerve hypoplasia occasionally may be associated with mental retardation, hypopituitarism, and absence of the septum pellucidum.

Papilledema

The name papilledema is reserved for swelling of the optic disk secondary to increased intracranial pressure. The name pseudopapilledema or elevated disk anomaly should be used for those cases of optic disk swelling due to other causes. Papilledema is a diagnosis that should be made with extreme caution. Because papilledema is a dynamic process, sometimes the diagnosis cannot be made on one examination, and serial observations must be made to record any progression.

The developmental sequence is an initial increase in the color of the disk, slight swelling of the veins, and blurring of the upper and lower edges of the disk. The hyperemic appearance of the disk is due to dilation of the smaller vessels. After a variable period of time, the upper, lower, and nasal margins become completely blurred, but the temporal margin often is still visible. The central cup begins to disappear, and the venous turgescence increases so that the veins are dark and tortuous. Small linear or splinter hemorrhages and cotton-wool spots due to infarction of the nerve fiber layer in the neighborhood of the disk often can be seen at this time. In the course of another week or 10 days the edges become more completely obscured, the central cup disappears, and the disk becomes more hyperemic due to the appearance of a number of tiny vessels on the surface.

It is important to remember that vision is almost never decreased in papilledema unless secondary optic atrophy has occurred in long-standing cases or macular changes have taken place. Fleeting obscurations or alterations in vision in one or both eyes may occur that last only a few seconds; they often are related to changes in posture. Visual field testing shows an enlarged blind spot and, in later cases, concentric constriction of the visual field. Regular visual field testing should be performed in all patients with long-standing papilledema, as it may give the first indication of beginning optic atrophy.

Causes of Optic Disk Edema

BRAIN TUMORS

Brain tumors with increased intracranial pressure (cerebrospinal fluid pressure must be above 200 mm H_2O) can cause optic disk edema. Approximately 80 percent of brain tumors are associated with papilledema, and tumors below the tentorium are more likely to produce it than tumors above the tentorium. Papilledema is rare in infants before the sutures close, as the skull enlarges to provide sufficient decompression to protect the nerves. In craniostenosis, where the sutures close early, even the growth of a normal brain can cause papilledema.

OTHER INTRACRANIAL CAUSES

Benign intracranial hypertension, meningitis, brain abscess, and prolonged seizures are other intracranial causes of papilledema.

LOCAL OCULAR PROBLEMS

Local ocular problems, such as uveitis or hypotony, and orbital disease (tumors or dysthyroid exophthalmos) can cause disk swelling

SYSTEMIC DISORDERS

Systemic disorders such as hypertension, blood dyscrasias, lead poisoning, pulmonary disease, i.e., Pickwickian syndrome, severe enough to cause a rise on P_{CO_2} and a fall in P_{O_2} are additional causes of disk edema.

PAPILLITIS

Papillitis occurs when an inflammatory or demyelinating process involves the visible optic nerve. Associated with disk swelling are an acute decrease in vision, a central scotoma on visual field examination, markedly reduced color vision, and an afferent pupillary defect. Papillitis is most frequently unilateral.

LEBER'S OPTIC NEUROPATHY

Leber's optic neuropathy is a sex-linked recessive disorder seen in young males between the ages of 15 and 20 years. In this condition there is profound bilateral visual loss and a swollen hyperemic appearance of each disk due to telangiectasia of the small blood vessels on the disk and peripapillary retina. No leakage of dye is seen on fluorescein angiography.

DRUSEN

Drusen of the optic nerve, one of the most common causes of benign disk edema in childhood, has already been discussed.

Optic Atrophy

The optic nerve in premature and full-term infants is pink or slightly pale. This occasional pallor should not be confused with optic atrophy, which implies a change in the function as well as the appearance of the optic nerve. Optic atrophy may be congenital, primary, secondary, glaucomatous, or consecutive.

Congenital optic atrophy is rare, and the diagnosis is made by exclusion and by the family history.

Primary optic atrophy is the most common type. The disk is stark white, the margins are sharply demarcated, the number of small vessels crossing the disk is reduced, and there is no elevation. Any process that compresses or stretches the nerve, obstructs its blood supply, or directly involves the nerve, such as demyelination, will cause primary optic atrophy.

Secondary optic atrophy follows prolonged untreated papilledema or papillitis. Secondary gliosis and mesenchymal reaction cause the characteristic dusky gray appearance of the disk. The margins are indistinct, and there may be some elevation of the nerve due to filling in of the physiologic cup.

Consecutive or ascending optic atrophy follows degeneration of the axons of the ganglion cells. Retinitis pigmentosa, extensive chorioretinitis, and other generalized disorders of retinal function are common causes and are usually obvious on fundus examination.

NYSTAGMUS

Nystagmus is defined as rhythmic involuntary oscillation of one or both eyes in any or all fields of gaze that occurs independently of the normal eye movements. Properly interpreted, it may be an extremely helpful diagnostic sign. Much of our confusion regarding nystagmus springs from our poor knowledge of its underlying neural basis and from the fact that different authors classify it in different ways. Not all forms of nystagmus fit into a neat classification; the following outline is presented as a general guide to the evaluation of such patients. It is not all-inclusive; rather, it concentrates on the types of nystagmus that have specific localizing value or are clinically useful.

Certain initial clinical observations are helpful in the final interpretation of nystagmus. Is the nystagmus pendular or jerk, horizontal, vertical, or rotary? It is monocular, binocular, or dissociated (different in each eye)? Observe the eyes for several minutes at close range and at a distance and note the effects of lateral and vertical gaze on the nystagmus. The direction of the nystagmus is named according to the direction of the fast phase, which is the easiest to see. Thus vestibular nystagmus to the right means that the fast phase of the nystagmus is to the right. The rate may be slow (10–40 beats/min), medium (40–100 beats/min), or fast (> 100 beats/min). The amplitude may be fine (a range of < 5°), moderate (a range of 5–15 degrees), or coarse (a range > 15°). The severity of the nystagmus is classified as grade I, II, or III. First-degree nystagmus is present on conjugate gaze to one side only; second-degree nystagmus is present on conjugate gaze to one side and straight ahead; third-degree nystagmus is present on conjugate gaze to both sides and straight ahead.

Nystagmus may occur in normal individuals; thus it is useful to separate it into physiologic and pathologic types.

Physiologic Nystagmus

VOLUNTARY NYSTAGMUS

Voluntary nystagmus differs from pathologic nystagmus in that the oscillations are of low amplitude, have extremely rapid rates, and cannot be maintained for more than a few minutes. It normally requires great concentration and probably some convergence. This harmless finding is seen occasionally in normal individuals, and it is considered to be the ocular equivalent of shuddering or shivering. However, it may be displayed by patients with emotional disorders, leading the unwary physician to pursue an unwarranted investigation.

END-POINT NYSTAGMUS

End-point nystagmus is a fine low-amplitude nystagmus commonly seen in normal patients, but only if they are required to look beyond the limit of binocular fixation. The fast phase is in the direction of gaze. The nystagmus disappears when the eyes are released from the extremes of gaze.

OPTOKINETIC NYSTAGMUS

With optokinetic nystagmus (OKN) an optokinetic tape or drum employing alternate black and white squares, stripes, or pictures will elicit a slow pursuit movement (initiated by the occipital lobe) and a rapid corrective saccade (initiated by the frontal lobe) in the opposite direction to refixate the next target. OKN responses are useful in the following clinical situations:

OKN responses may be elicited in the infant at the time fixation reflexes have developed, about the third or fourth month. An intact OKN response implies visual acuity of about 20/400, which is about the level of visual acuity to be expected in a child at the age of 4 months. At age 1 year, the expected visual acuity would be in the region of 20/200; at age 2 years, in the region of 20/40; at age 3 years, in the region of 20/30.

An intact monocular OKN response may be a helpful confirmatory sign in an emotionally disturbed child who claims severely reduced vision or absence of vision in one eye.

The OKN response is occasionally helpful in localizing a lesion causing complete homonymous hemianopia. Such a defect with normal horizontal OKN response suggests a vascular lesion in the occipital lobe, whereas such hemianopia with absence of OKN responses when directing the stimulus toward the side of the lesion suggests a mass lesion extending into the parietal lobe.

A vertical OKN response with the stripes rotating downward is a quick and simple method to accentuate convergence retraction nystagmus seen as part of Parinaud's syndrome.

The OKN may be helpful in patients with congenital nystagmus. If no horizontal OKN response can be superimposed, but there is a normal vertical OKN response, a relatively good prognosis can be made. If it is impossible to superimpose a horizontal or vertical OKN response in a child with congenital nystagmus, the visual prognosis is much less favorable.

Pathologic Nystagmus

PENDULAR NYSTAGMUS

Pendular nystagmus, also called sensory or ocular nystagmus, is a disorder in which the rates of oscillation are approximately the same in both directions. The nystagmus is almost invariably horizontal, and on conjugate gaze to either side it frequently is converted to a jerk-type nystagmus, with the fast component toward the side of gaze. This type of nystagmus is most often encountered in patients with defective central vision from infancy. The etiology may be obvious, as in congenital cataracts, bilateral macular scars, and optic atrophy, or subtle, as in albinism or total color blindness. In general, the greater the visual defect, the more irregular and more coarse the ocular oscillation. The development of a normal saccadic mechanism seems to depend on the preservation of normal central vision from birth. Macular impulses provide positional sense for the eyes. In the absence of central vision, this positional information is lacking, and pendular nystagmus occurs. Binocular loss of vision that develops before the age of 2 years almost always results in pendular nystagmus; loss of binocular vision after 6 years of age never results in nystagmus. With loss of binocular vision between 2 and 6 years of age, the development of nystagmus is variable.

SPASMUS NUTANS

Spasmus nutans is a special type of pendular nystagmus in which the oscillations are characteristically rapid and often asymmetric in the two eyes. It may be entirely monocular, and it is the most common cause of unilateral horizontal nystagmus in childhood. Head nodding often accompanies the nystagmus, and occasionally there is torticollis; but all three characteristics are not invariably present. It is not associated with organic disease, and no treatment is indicated; the condition is self-limited, with complete recovery in 1–2 years. It has been suggested that the condition results from delayed maturation of the mechanism for coordination of ocular and head movements.

SEESAW NYSTAGMUS

Seesaw nystagmus is characterized by elevation and intorsion of one eye, with depression and extorsion of the other eye. A bitemporal visual field defect should be sought, as this condition is classically seen with parachiasmal lesions, but it also has been described in patients with vascular and demyelinating disease involving the brain stem.

JERK NYSTAGMUS

Jerk nystagmus (also called motor nystagmus) is characterized by unequal velocities in the two directions of oscillation. Thus a slow component in one direction is followed by a rapid return to the original position. The direction of the nystagmus is named for the faster of the two components. The nystagmus is ususally horizontal, occasionally rotary, but never vertical. It is usually noted at birth or shortly thereafter; it is transmitted in a sex-linked recessive or rarely dominant fashion. A neutral point in which the nystagmus slows or stops is often seen. Head nodding or head turning may indicate an effort to place the eyes in this position of least nystagmus, where visual acuity may be normal or near normal. Convergence may slow or stop the nystagmus. An important clinical point to remember is that congenital jerk nystagmus is horizontal in all fields of gaze.

LATENT NYSTAGMUS

Latent nystagmus may be revealed by covering one eye or by increasing the brightness contrast between the two eyes. Visual acuity often is seriously reduced with one eye covered, but it is normal with both eyes open. The fast phase of the nystagmus is toward the uncovered eye. It is frequently associated with strabismus. The importance of latent nystagmus lies in the fact that it labels the nystagmus as congenital in origin and not of neurologic significance.

PERIPHERAL VESTIBULAR NYSTAGMUS

Peripheral vestibular nystagmus is produced by lesions affecting the eighth nerve or the labyrinth. The direction of the slow component is always in the direction of flow of endolymph in the semicircular canal, and the fast component (by which the nystagmus is named) will be opposite the flow. The nystagmus may be horizontal, rotary, or jerk, with the fast component directed away from a destructive lesion and toward the side of an irritative lesion. It may only be present with the head in a particular field of gaze. It is usually associated with vertigo, tinnitus, and decreased hearing. The nystagmus and vertigo usually are short-lived.

CENTRAL VESTIBULAR NYSTAGMUS

Central vestibular nystagmus is due to disease of the lateral or medial vestibular nuclei or their connections with the cerebellum or brain stem. The nystagmus is also horizontal or rotary, but tinnitus and vertigo are usually mild or absent. Barbiturates, Dilantin, and Streptomycin are among the drugs that may cause toxic vestibular nystagmus.

BRUNS NYSTAGMUS

Bruns nystagmus is a gaze-evoked type of nystagmus with a coarse, slow nystagmus in one direction and a faster, small-amplitude nystagmus in the other. It is seen in patients with mass lesions, such as an acoustic neuroma compressing the cerebellum or pontine tegmentum on the side of the slower nystagmus.

GAZE-EVOKED NYSTAGMUS

Gaze-evoked nystagmus is one of the most common types of nystagmus and the least helpful in terms of anatomic localization. It implies a structural or chemical abnormality of the conjugate gaze center in the brain stem, but it also may be seen when looking in the field of action of a paretic extraocular muscle. A Tensilon test to rule out myasthenia gravis should be done in all such patients.

INTERNUCLEAR OPHTHALMOPLEGIA

Internuclear ophthalmoplegia (INO) is a classic example of gaze-evoked nystagmus due to a lesion of the median longitudinal fasciculus. This consists of paresis of the medial rectus during adduction of one eye and a coarse horizontal nystagmus of the abducting fellow eye. The ability of the medial rectus to function on convergence is frequently intact. The most common cause of bilateral INO is demyelinating disease, whereas unilateral INO is seen in demyelinating or vascular lesions affecting the brain stem. In childhood it may be the presenting sign of a pontine glioma, and it has also been reported in myasthenia gravis (pseudo INO).

VERTICAL NYSTAGMUS

Vertical nystagmus in the primary position is always abnormal, whereas vertical nystagmus in upward gaze is commonly seen in drug intoxications, such as with barbiturates and Dilantin.

Coarse, large-amplitude upbeat nystagmus (fast component of the nystagmus is up), when present in the primary position, increasing on upgaze and decreasing on downgaze, is seen in lesions involving the anterior vermis of the cerebellum.

Small-amplitude upbeat nystagmus in the primary position is usually seen as a consequence of medullary infarctions.

In downbeat nystagmus the fast phase of the nystagmus is down and often is accentuated in the down and lateral position of gaze. Oscillopsia, illusory movement of objects, is a frequent complaint. This condition is usually seen with anomalies of the cranial cervical junction, such as platybasia or the Arnold-Chiari malformation, with secondary compression of the medulla, upper cervical cord; or lower end of the cerebellum.

PERIODIC ALTERNATING NYSTAGMUS

Periodic alternating nystagmus is a rare form of nystagmus that points to a low medullary or cranial cervical junction lesion. It may be missed if the eyes are not observed for a period of a few minutes or more. There is a gradual increase in the amplitude of the nystagmus (which is horizontal or horizontal-rotary jerk type) over a period of 1–3 min. The amplitude then gradually decreases, until a nystagmus-free interval of up to 30 sec. is seen. Nystagmus to the opposite side then follows, again lasting 1–3 min, and the cycle is then continuously repeated.

CONVERGENCE RETRACTION NYSTAGMUS

Convergence retraction nystagmus is seen as part of the sylvian aqueduct syndrome, along with paresis of upward gaze and light–near dissociation of the pupil. Pronounced spasmodic retraction of the globes occurs on attempted upgaze. It localizes the lesion to the tectum of the midbrain, and in childhood it is commonly the result of a pineal tumor or midbrain glioma. It may be demonstrated most easily by means of the OKN drum with the stripes rotating downward.

DISSOCIATED NYSTAGMUS

Dissociated nystagmus designates nystagmus that may be vertical, horizontal, or rotary and simultaneously different in the two eyes, or significantly greater in one eye than the other. It may be seen in amblyopia, spasmus nutans, or internuclear ophthalmoplegia; but it may be a sign of cerebellar or brain-stem disease. When associated with posterior fossa lesions, the nystagmus may be vertical in one eye and horizontal or rotary in the other; it is then frequently associated with oscillopsia and ataxia.

NYSTAGMUSLIKE CONDITIONS

Nystagmus-like conditions may superficially resemble nystagmus, but they are not commonly classified as such.

Oculomotor apraxia. In oculomotor apraxia, which is most commonly seen in young males, there is retention of involuntary lateral versions, but there is failure to initiate voluntary movements on command or in response to a visual stimulus. The most striking feature of the condition is a compensatory purposeful headthrust with an overshoot of the eyes beyond the object of regard, usually with a blink to break fixation. The headthrusts beyond the object are necessary because the vestibular stimulation induced causes deviation of the eyes opposite the direction of the desired gaze. With full lateral rotation of the head, however, the eyes are brought into the line of fixation. Once this is achieved, the head gradually moves back until the positions of the head and eyes again become normal. The etiology of the condition is generally regarded as benign if there is no evidence of neurological disease, but its association in two cases of cerebellar medulloblastoma has been reported.

Ocular bobbing. A brisk conjugate downward movement of the eyes is followed by a slow drift up to the point of fixation, with a frequency of 2–12 beats/min. There is associated paralysis of horizontal conjugate gaze. In adults it is generally the result of severe vascular disease affecting the pons; in the pediatric age group it usually implies a large neoplastic pontine lesion.

Ocular dysmetria. Conjugate overshooting (or rarely undershooting) of the eyes is noted when gaze is shifted from an eccentric lateral position to an object directly in front of the patient. Subsequent fine refixation movements serve to bring the object of regard onto fixation.

Ocular flutter. Bursts of rapid horizontal oscillation lasting for only a few seconds occur spontaneously or with changes in fixation.

Opsoclonus. Constant chaotic and conjugate eye movements both vertically and horizontally occur and persist during sleep. There frequently are myoclonic movements of the face, arms, or legs. The disorder usually follows an attack of benign encephalitis, but it may be associated with the presence of an occult neuroblastoma, and this condition must be specifically excluded in a child with opsoclonus.

All three conditions (dysmetria, flutter, and opsoclonus) are the results of a disorder of the cerebellum or the cerebellar connections in the brain stem. It has been postulated that the three conditions result from progressive disruption of the precise control of saccadic eye movements by the cerebellum.

Spasm of the near reflex. This functional disorder of gaze is not uncommon in children and often is confused with a bilateral sixth nerve palsy. It is especially noted when attention is diverted to the eyes; it consists of spastic overaction of each of the three components of the near reflex: accommodation, convergence, and miosis. These patients complain of blurred vision because the accommodative spasm causes induced myopia. Convergence on attempted lateral gaze produces the picture of a sixth nerve palsy, but it can be differentiated from this by the miosis that accompanies the accommodation.

THE PUPIL

Light Reflex Pathway

The afferent arc of the light reflex pathway begins with stimulation of the rods and cones within the retina. Impulses pass along the optic nerve, decussate at the chiasm in a fashion similar to the visual afferent fibers, and pass to the posterior third of the optic tract. Here the pupillary fibers branch away just before the lateral geniculate body and pass through the brachium of the superior colliculus to the pretectum, where they synapse at the pretectal nucleus. Postsynaptic fibers hemidecussate around the periaqueductal gray and provide equal innervation to each Edinger-Westphal (EW) nucleus. The oculomotor nerve carries the efferent outflow fibers from the EW nucleus through the midbrain and cerebral peduncles, into the interpeduncular space along the base of the brain, through the cavernous sinus, and into the orbit via the superior orbital fissure. These parasympathetic fibers travel with the nerves to the inferior oblique and give off a short motor route to the ciliary ganglion. Postsynaptic fibers are carried by the short ciliary nerve to the pupillary sphincter. The pupillary fibers are presumed to travel superficially along the oculomotor nerve; thus they are vulnerable to compression and often are spared in microvascular infarctions of the oculomotor nerve in diabetes mellitus.

Sympathetic Pathway

The sympathetic pathway that innervates the iris dilator muscle is conveniently divided by the synapses into three sections:

Central.   Fibers originate in the posterior hypothalamus and descend in the ventrolateral portion of the brain stem and spinal cord through the ciliospinal center of Budge, where they synapse at the C-8/T-2 level.

Preganglionic.   At the C-8/T-2 level in the spinal cord, preganglionic fibers leave and travel up the sympathetic chain to synapse in the superior cervical ganglion.

Postganglionic.   From the superior cervical ganglion, postganglionic fibers accompany the carotid artery to the gasserian ganglion of the fifth cranial nerve. There they enter the orbit via the ophthalmic division of the trigeminal to the ciliary ganglion and onto the long ciliary nerve to the eye.

Near Reflex Pathway

Accommodation, convergence, and miosis are the three components of the near reflex. All are mediated through the oculomotor complex, and they faciliate clear vision when objects are brought close to the eyes. The afferent arc arises in the medial rectus muscles and travels in the third nerve or the ophthalmic division of the fifth nerve to the mesencephalic root of the fifth nerve. From there a relay is made to the convergence center and to the EW nucleus. The efferent arc travels down the third cranial nerve. The stimulus to the EW nucleus associated with a near vision effort thus takes a more ventral path than that serving the light reflex.

Normal Findings

The pupils of premature infants may not react well, and they are difficult to dilate. The pupils of full-term infants are slightly miotic, but pupillary reactions are present, if a little less extensive than those of adolescence. Up to the age of 3–4 years, anisocoria (inequality in diameters of pupils) may be present in normal infants, and this is considered normal if the pupillary reactions are unimpaired. Pupillary unrest is seen in all normal individuals. This constant state of motion of the pupil represents dynamic equilibrium of sympathetic and parasympathetic innervation. When the pupillary excursions exceed those of normal physiologic pupillary unrest, the condition is called hippus. Neither condition has any pathologic significance.

Examination of the Pupil

The examination should be carried out in a dimly lit room, and accommodation should be controlled at all times by having the patient fixate on a distant object. The face is illuminated from below with a bright handlight, and both pupil size and interpalpebral fissures are measured directly with a millimeter rule. Clinical observation of an abnormal pupil should be tabulated in the following manner:

1. Room light
2. Dim light
3. Direct light response
4. Consensual light response: Is an afferent pupil defect present?
5. Near response
6. Slit-lamp reaction
7. Drug reactions

Examination of the pupils in bright illumination accentuates the anisocoria of a third nerve lesion, whereas examination of the pupils in dim light accentuates the anisocoria seen as part of Horner's syndrome. Remember to compare the amplitude of the near response with that of the light response. A slit-lamp examination may show the presence of trauma to the iris sphincter or vermiform movements of the iris sphincter that occur as part of Adie's syndrome.

Congenital Pupil Abnormalities

Aniridia. Absence of the iris (usually incomplete) is transmitted as a dominant characteristic, and frequently it is associated with secondary glaucoma, cataracts, nystagmus, macular hypoplasia, and mental retardation. These relationships are described in more detail in other chapters.

It is especially important to remember that a child with aniridia with no family history of the disorder should be watched carefully for the development of Wilms' tumor. Male children under 3 years of age with genital abnormalities or mental retardation are particularly at risk.

Iris coloboma. Iris coloboma results from incomplete closure of the fetal fissure and causes a defect of the iris, usually below and nasally. It is often associated with other developmental defects, particularly subnormal mentality.

Ectopic pupils. Usually the displacement is up and out from the center of the cornea. There may be associated displacement of the lens and congenital glaucoma.

Persistent pupillary membranes. These threadlike bands run across the pupillary aperture and attach to the lesser circle of the iris. They are remnants of the embryonic pupillary membrane, and they rarely cause any visual symptoms. Occasionally there may be an associated anterior capsular cataract.

Heterochromia. In heterochromia the iris of one eye differs in color from the iris of the other. It may be simple heterochromia, where one eye is gray and the other brown, with no associated ocular pathology. The lighter eye is the pathologic eye in congenital Horner's syndrome, Fuchs' heterochromic cyclitis, and iris atrophy. The darker eye is abnormal in melanocytosis, siderosis, and diffuse iris melanoma.

Important Pathologic Pupillary Reactions

AMAUROTIC PUPILLARY REACTION

In amaurotic pupillary reaction the pupillary responses of a patient with an absolutely blind eye will be the following: no direct light response in the blind eye; no consensual response in the fellow eye; intact direct response in the normal eye; intact consensual response in the blind eye.

AFFERENT PUPIL DEFECT

Afferent pupil defects are also called Marcus Gun pupils and are demonstrated by the swinging flashlight test. Both pupils constrict if the light is shone in the normal eye; but if the light is then moved quickly to the affected eye, both pupils dilate (Fig. 6–15). It is the most valuable of all the pupillary tests and is an extremely sensitive indicator of even subtle impairment of optic nerve function. It is particularly useful in the diagnosis of retrobulbar neuritis or optic nerve tumor when the disk appears normal. It is best done in a semidarkened room with a bright handlight.

LIGHT-NEAR DISSOCIATION

Light–near dissocation implies a pupillary near reaction that is greater than the light reaction; it is a useful concept to remember in evaluating pupillary reactions. Light–near dissociation of the pupils is seen in a lesion involving the pretectal area of the upper midbrain (e.g., pincaloma) that interferes with the pupillary light reflex pathway. The pupils are dilated and do not react to light, but they react briskly to near stimuli (Fig. 6–16). The near reaction is not involved, as the near reflex pathway is more ventrally located in the midbrain. Gliomas of the quadrigeminal plate, encephalitis, and vascular disease have been reported as causing light–near dissociation. Frequently the pupillary findings are seen together with failure of upward gaze and retraction nystagmus as part of Parinaud's syndrome.

ARGYLL ROBERTSON PUPILS

Argyll Robertson Pupils are irregular and miotic and may be unequal. They do not react to light, despite near-normal visual acuity, but they respond well to near stimuli (Fig. 6–17). The defect is most likely in the midbrain; it is almost pathognomonic of syphilis, but it can also be found in diabetes mellitus.

EFFERENT DEFECTS

Preganglionic lesions. Preganglionic lesions (Hutchinson's pupil) involve herniation of the temporal lobe and compression of the third nerve

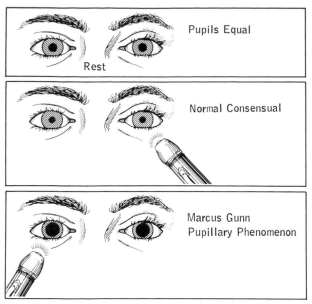

Figure 6-15. Marcus Gunn phenomenon. Pupils are equal when at rest. A normal direct and consensual reaction is noted when a light is directed in the normal eye. When the light is briskly moved to the affected eye, both pupils dilate.

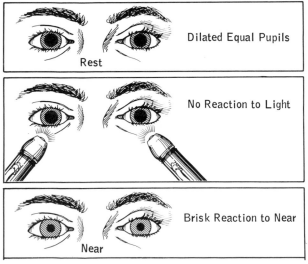

Figure 6-16. Light–near dissociation. Parinaud's syndrome. Both pupils are dilated and nonreactive to light, but they have a brisk reaction to near stimuli.

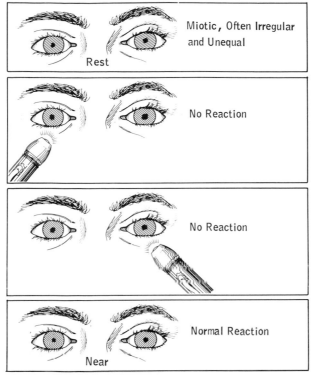

Rest — Miotic, Often Irregular and Unequal

No Reaction

No Reaction

Near — Normal Reaction

Figure 6-17. Light–near dissociation. Argyll Robertson pupils. Pupils are miotic and irregular, with no reaction to light in either eye, but having a normal reaction to near stimuli.

against the petroclinoid ligament, causing a dilated pupil on the ipsilateral side. This pupillary reaction is a reliable indicator of the side of an expanding mass such as a subdural hematoma (Fig. 6–18).

Postganglionic lesions. Postganglionic lesions (Adie's tonic pupil) are usually unilateral; they are more common in females and occasionally are seen in teenagers. The pupil is dilated and reacts sluggishly or not at all to light. Characteristically, a slow tonic redilation following contraction to a near target is seen. Slit-lamp examination confirms this slow tonic reaction to light and frequently shows vermiform (wormlike) movements of the iris sphincter under illumination. Weak solutions of pilocarpine (e.g., 0.1 percent) will constrict the pupil because of denervation hypersensitivity (Fig. 6–19).

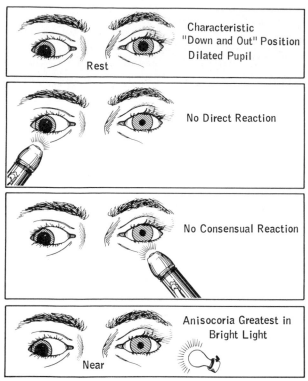

Figure 6-18.   Right third nerve palsy. (The right lid has been elevated.) The pupil is dilated, with no reaction to light or near stimuli. The pupillary inequality is greatest in bright illumination.

FIXED DILATED PUPIL

The patient with a fixed dilated pupil presents a common emergency room dilemma. Paralytic mydriasis due to an early third nerve palsy or an Adie's pupil can be separated from the more common pharmacologic mydriasis due to inadvertent instillation of atropine-like drugs. The pupil that is dilated secondary to instillation of mydriatic drops will fail to construct to pilocarpine 0.5 percent or 1 percent.

HORNER'S SYNDROME

The classic triad of ptosis, miosis, and absence of sweating on the ipsilateral side of the face is seen in Horner's syndrome (Fig. 6–20). The responses of the miotic pupil to both light and near stimuli are normal. It is most often seen in childhood as a result of birth injury to the brachial plexus.

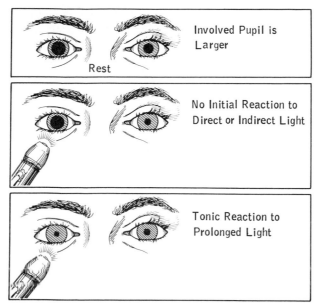

Figure 6-19.   Adie's tonic pupil. The right pupil is larger, with a
slow tonic reaction to prolonged light, and a slow tonic redilation
following constriction to light.

Heterochromia is seen in congenital Horner's syndrome because lack of sympathetic influence on the melanocytes of the iris results in a lighter iris on the
involved side. The diagnosis can be made clinically, but pharmacologic drug
testing may confirm the diagnosis and localize the site of the lesion.

Cocaine (10 percent) will fail to dilate all Horner's syndrome pupils and
is useful for confirming the diagnosis but not for localizing the lesion.

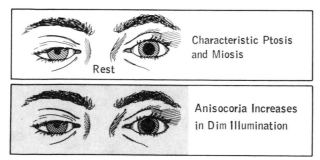

Figure 6-20.   Horner's syndrome. The right pupil is miotic, the
pupillary inequality is greatest in dim illumination.

Paredrine (1 percent) will dilate all normal pupils and the miotic pupil of Horner's syndrome unless it is caused by a postganglionic lesion. Paredrine releases norepinephine from the postganglionic presynaptic vesicles and therefore causes pupillary dilation only if third-order neurons are intact.

Stephen S. Feman, M.D.

7

Disorders of the Retina, Vitreous, and Choroid

PATIENT EXAMINATION

The most important feature in clinical evaluation is adequate visualization of the retina, vitreous, and choroid. This requires maximal dilation in a cooperative patient.

The common topical medications used for dilation are potent anticholinergic agents. Injudicious use of such drugs can produce systemic levels that are within the toxic range. In some instances the topical medication may flow into the nasolacrimal duct with the tears, and the portion that is not absorbed by the mucous membranes will be swallowed with the saliva; in other cases a near-lethal dose may be absorbed directly through the conjunctiva. For these reasons it is imperative to specify the concentration of medication and the details of the delivery method.[1,2]

With awareness of these risks, the following drug combination has been found to be most successful; it has permitted examinations to include the retina from the optic nerve to the ora serrata, the pars plana, and the posterior border of the ciliary body, as well as the total vitreous body. The combination of medications used for a detailed retinal examination consists of one drop of 2.5 percent phenylephrine ophthalmic solution followed by one drop of 1.0 percent cyclopentolate ophthalmic solution followed by one more drop of 2.5 percent phenylephrine ophthalmic solution. Each drop is placed on the lower conjunctival surface while the lower eyelid is retracted; the lid is allowed to return to its normal position against the globe, and the excess drop and tears are wiped dry with cotton. After 1 min the second drop is applied in a similar manner; 1 min later the third drop is applied. Maximal dilation occurs within 30 min. It is strongly recommended that when it is not necessary to evaluate fine retinal detail, medications of less toxicity be used.[1,2]

A cooperative adult is less than comfortable during a detailed retinal examination; it would be surprising to find a pediatric patient any more at ease in a similar situation. However, if a good doctor–patient relationship can be established, the child may permit the examination. Except in the neonatal population, a complete retinal and vitreal examination of a restrained patient has been found to be an unsatisfactory technique. For this reason the use of sedation and the assistance of a pediatric anesthesiologist may be required.

An analysis of the various methods of inspecting the retina is beyond the scope of this chapter. However, it is important to be aware that there are techniques adaptable specifically for a pediatric examination. The direct ophthalmoscope produces a magnified view of the posterior pole of the eye; this permits detailed examination of the optic nerve and the retina posterior to the ocular equator. The binocular indirect ophthalmoscope can be used ot obtain a stereoscopic view of these same areas; however, it is common to combine this with a scleral indentation technique that allows the examination to be extended to include the anterior retina and posterior ciliary body. Additional information can be obtained with the use of the slit-lamp biomicroscope and contact lens. Permanent records of ocular findings may be produced by drawings, fundus photography with fluorescein angiography, qualitative and quantitative ocular ultrasonography, and electroretinography. In most cases it would be inappropriate to recommend therapy or genetic counseling without the basic clinical data obtained by these tests.

RETINAL AND VITREAL VASCULAR DISORDERS

Retrolental Fibroplasia

Retrolental fibroplasia is a retinovascular disorder that is related, in most cases, to oxygen exposure. The association between the increased incidence of retrolental fibroplasia and the duration of oxygen exposure has been well documented. However, not all patients treated with oxygen develop this disorder; retrolental fibroplasia has been reported in patients who have had no oxygen exposure, and closely matched patients treated identically do not always develop similar problems. Therefore, although oxygen is a major factor in this disorder, additional features that are still unknown may contribute substantially to its development.[3,4]

The phases of this disorder have been divided into stages of clinical activity and grades of residual scarring:

Stage I: dilated and tortuous retinal vessels without neovascularization.
Stage II: neovascularization of the retinal periphery.
Stage III: less than one quadrant of tractional retinal detachment.
Stage IV: more than one quadrant of tractional retinal detachment.
Stage V: retinal detachment involving all quadrants.

Spontaneous regression has been reported in many patients in stage I and stage II. Experimental surgical procedures have been devised for patients in stages II and III. In this population anatomic surgical success is not rare, but the complication rate is too high to warrant routine surgical intervention when a chance for spontaneous regression exists.

Grade I: abnormal retinal vessels and fibrous tissue on the peripheral retinal surface.

Grade II: small areas of localized retinal detachment.

Grade III: distortion of the optic nerve and a retinal fold extending from the optic nerve to the retinal periphery.

Grade IV: retrolental tissue encroaching the pupil, but some residual attached retina present.

Grade V: total pupillary obstruction, with no attached retina.

There is still controversy regarding the role of the ophthalmologist in the care of these patients. Nevertheless, the following guide may be of value to mediate the clinical conflicts:

1. It is inappropriate for an ophthalmologist to recommend changes in oxygen therapy. The pediatrician is using the smallest concentration and duration of oxygen compatible with the life of the patient.

2. The stages and grades described previously are of interest, but they can be a source of confusion. It is always better to describe in detail what is seen in the eye.

3. There is no known therapy that can reverse this disorder in a reliable and reproducible manner. However, some of its complications, such as retinal detachment, can be treated successfully. It is the role of the physician to counsel the family in regard to the overall care of the child with this visual problem.

4. When the disorder is progressing, frequent examinations are needed to ascertain its final outcome. It is not uncommon for these examinations to be performed at biweekly or monthly intervals for a period of 6 months or more. If the disorder ceases to progress at any stage or grade less than V, repetitive examinations are needed because of the high incidence of rhegmatogenous retinal detachments in these patients. Corrective surgery for this latter development is successful in some cases.

5. If the earliest signs of retrolental fibroplasia are not present at the time of discharge from the nursery, they are rarely demonstrable at a later date.

Persistent Hyperplastic Primary Vitreous

Persistent hyperplastic primary vitreous usually appears as a uniocular disorder in full-term infants. Primary vitreous is an opaque vascularized tissue derived in part from embryologic mesoderm. Usually it starts to disappear when the embryo is at the 26-mm stage, about the sixth week of gestation. The vitreous that replaces the primary vitreous is optically clear, and this substitution is complete before birth. Persistent hyperplastic primary vitreous may be present in any portion of the ocular vitreous cavity. However, it is most frequently noted adjacent to the lens in the area occupied during embryologic development by the tunica vasculosa lentis.

The clinical findings noted in the most common form of persistent hyperplastic primary vitreous consist of a retrolental neovascularized mass in an eye with relative microphthalmia (Fig. 7-1). This neovascularization grows onto the lens and can produce hemorrhage into the lens. The recurring episodes of hemorrhage and inflammation are associated with destruction of the anterior segment of the eye. This may result in a blind and painful eye that requires enucleation. In many cases this development can be prevented by surgically removing the primary vitreous. However, because of the optical problems associated with microphthalmia, good visual results are uncommon.[3]

Coats' Disorder

Coats' disorder was originally described between the years 1908 and 1912. A modern interpretation includes at least three different retinal disorders: type I, a subretinal exudation in which one must assume the existence of an underlying vascular anomaly, although one is unable to demonstrate it with clinical techniques; type II, a combination of small blood vessel abnormalities and subretinal exudation; type III, a large retinal angioma. Retinal angiography permits easy definition of these pathologic forms. Type I is reported rarely in the pediatric population. Type III is the ocular angioma of von Hippel in the von Hippel-Lindau syndrome. Type II is a characteristic pediatric ophthalmic syndrome consisting of telangiectasia, dilated capillary aneurysms, and eosinophilic PAS-positive exudate located in the outer retina.[6]

Coats' disorder of type II is most frequently noted as a uniocular problem in male children (Fig. 7–2). The area of the intraretinal edema and subretinal exudate may increase, although spontaneous regression and resolution have been reported in some cases. Any form of therapy that can destroy the underlying pathology can be of benefit for these patients. In recent years argon laser photocoagulation has been the most popular treatment modality.

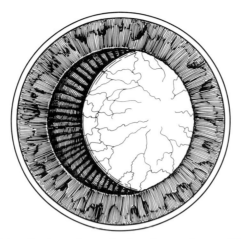

Figure 7-1. Persistent hyperplastic primary vitreous. The lens is dislocated, and the ciliary processes are being pulled up by the vascular membrane, which can be seen through the lens.

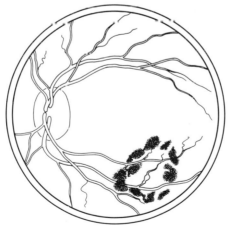

Figure 7-2. Coats' disorder. Retinal telangiectasia with edema and exudates.

MALIGNANT TUMORS

Retinoblastoma

Retinoblastoma is the most common primary intraocular malignant tumor in children. It is reported once in every 25,000 births in the United States. The genetic pattern associated with this tumor implies autosomal dominant heredity; however, more than 90 percent of cases may represent spontaneous mutations arising in the affected individual. For these reasons the tumor survivors are most benefited by genetic counseling.

Tumor is present in both eyes in over 30 percent of involved individuals. The tumor is multicentric; that is, there is often more than one site of primary tumor in an individual eye. The tumor can arise in any retinal layer; those that originate near the vitreoretinal surface and grow into the vitreous are called endophytic, and those that arise near the choroid and grow into the subretinal space are called exophytic.

Retinoblastomas are usually cheesy white in color; blood vessels may grow within and on the surface of these tumors. Small tumor "seeds" can grow as independent islands floating freely in the vitreous. Sharply demarcated, glistening white calcifications appear on or within most tumors.

This tumor may present as an acute ocular inflammation. This is because the tumor outgrows its vascular supply and becomes necrotic. Usually this is noted in tumors that are outside of the visual axis. Those within the pupillary axis can cause strabismus and/or a white pupillary reflex that enable the diagnosis to be made at an earlier stage.

This is a highly malignant tumor capable of widespread metastasis. It may grow directly along the optic nerve into the brain. It can enter the vasculature via the choroid to spread hematogenously. It may invade the orbital lymphatics.

It has been estimated that less than 1 percent of cases undergo spontaneous regression. For this reason, many ophthalmologists recommend that a patient with uniocular disease and no metastases be treated by enucleation.

Although this is the most common intraocular primary tumor in children, most ophthalmologists refer these patients to centers that specialize in the treatment of this disorder. Antitumor therapy, without enucleation, is available at some of these medical centers. The following modalities have been used either alone or in combination: cryotherapy, photocoagulation, chemotherapy, and radiation therapy. In general, the visual prognosis for eyes that have been treated is related to the tumor grade at the time of treatment initiation:

Group I (very favorable): all tumors behind the ocular equator; all tumors smaller than four disk diameters in cross section.

Group II (favorable): all tumors behind the ocular equator; the largest tumor less than 10 disk diameters in size.

Group III (doubtful): any tumor anterior to the ocular equator; any solitary tumor greater than 10 disk diameters.

Group IV (unfavorable): any tumor reaching the ora serrata; multiple tumors, when some of them are larger than 10 disk diameters.

Group V (very unfavorable): massive tumors involving over half of the retina; vitreous seeding.[7]

Leukemias

The leukemias commonly involve the eyes in pediatric patients. Most frequently, retinal hemorrhages are noted. White lesions within the retina may represent degenerating nerve fibers or leukemic infiltrates. Although these retinal changes may be related to thrombocytopenia or anemia, the degree of retinopathy has not been found to have a statistical correlation with the leukemic prognosis.

Malignant Melanoma

Malignant melanoma of the choroid is quite rare in children. Malignant melanoma of the iris is described in another chapter.

RHEGMATOGENOUS RETINAL DETACHMENTS

Rhegmatogenous retinal detachments caused by breaks through the full thickness of the retina are uncommon in children. Trauma is the most frequent cause of this problem, which may account for the preponderance of cases in males. Although a penetrating wound may be an obvious cause, a retinal break can occur after minor blunt trauma that has no visible cutaneous bruise. In the latter situation the symptoms may be subtle and slow in development. The child may be unaware of the slowly progressing visual defect until months or years after the inciting incident.

In many cases the ocular trauma results in some degree of vitreous liquefaction; this fluid can percolate through the retinal break to detach the retina from the underlying tissues. In other patients the retinal break may be large enough to allow the more gelatinous vitreous to slide beneath the retina. Closure of the retinal hole and removal of the subretinal fluid produce visual improvement in most patients.[9]

Pediatric rhegmatogenous retinal detachment without trauma is not uncommon in patients with prematurity or myopia. However, an additional feature is reported with increasing frequency: a previously undiagnosed and partially regressed form of retrolental fibroplasia. These patients may have had spontaneously regressing stage II retrolental fibroplasia, as indicated by a history of prematurity and myopia and the presence of small tufts of fibrous tissue extending from the retina into the vitreous. Although this retinal detachment may not develop until the patient's teenage years, a careful review of the hospital records may reveal neonatal oxygen levels compatible with retrolental fibroplasia.

The surgical therapy of rhegmatogenous retinal detachment is beyond the scope of this chapter. However, it is important to emphasize that therapy does not end when the retina has been anatomically reattached. When the detachment is present, there is an anatomic cause of amblyopia; after the anatomic problem is corrected, antiamblyopia therapy is indicated until maximal visual improvement occurs.

DISORDERS OF INNER RETINAL LAYERS

There are several metabolic disorders that are noted for involvement of the inner retinal layers. The most frequent representative of this group is a disorder of sphingolipid metabolism known as Tay-Sachs disease. This disease is inherited in an autosomal recessive manner. Patients with this disorder are unable to metabolize ganglioside, which results in swelling and degeneration of ganglion cells throughout the central nervous system. Within the retina of a patient with Tay-Sachs disease the ganglion cells develop an opaque white color. There are no ganglion cells in the fovea; thus it appears as a cherry-red spot when contrasted with the adjacent white retina. The functional loss of retinal ganglion cells results in blindness in the first 2 years of life; the progressive functional loss of ganglion cells in the central nervous system results in paralysis and death.

The carrier state for this disorder does not have typical ocular or neurologic manifestations. However, a serum enzyme defect can be identified in all asymptomatic carriers. Genetic counseling is recommended for such patients.[10,11]

DEGENERATIONS OF OUTER RETINAL LAYERS

Several pediatric disorders involve the outer retinal layers. Some disorders are specific in that cells of a particular anatomic shape or functional variety are the only ones involved; other degenerations are more diffuse, and some degenerations have unknown histopathologic features and are classified in this group on the basis of presumptive clinical evidence. The cell-specific disorders are rare and will not be discussed.

Retinitis Pigmentosa

Retinitis pigmentosa is a name used to describe a common clinical manifestation of a group of degenerations that diffusely involve the outer retinal layers. At least 16 major disorders have this clinical manifestation.[12] Each of these disorders has a different metabolic and/or genetic defect. For this reason the following description will be limited to general features common to most of these disorders.

Retinal photoreceptor degeneration is the first sign of the disorder. However, in time, more widespread retinal degeneration and atrophy will occur. Glial tissue will replace some of the retinal cell loss. The retinal vessels will become narrow. The retinal pigment epithelium will become depigmented, and pigmentary tissue will be found adjacent to the vessels in the neurosensory retina. This ocular degeneration received the name that is historically associated with it, retinitis pigmentosa, from this pigmentary change. However, a modern understanding of the developing pathology indicates that pigmentary change is not a necessary part of the disorder, although it is frequently noted.

Almost all patients initially complain of night blindness. At such times a ring scotoma, representing degeneration of the equatorial retina, is noted. In these patients paravascular pigment deposits in a bone spicule pattern are noted in the peripheral retina (Fig. 7-3). A severe lack of intraretinal electrical activity, as measured by the electroretinogram, is a characteristic of these patients and is uncommon in other disorders. The diffuse retinal degeneration is associated with optic atrophy and loss of central vision in some forms of this disorder.

Vitelliform Macular Degeneration

Vitelliform macular degeneration is believed to involve the outer retinal layers, but histopathologic documentation is incomplete. Clinically this disorder appears as a yellow deposit of an egg-yolk color beneath the retina in the macular area (Fig. 7-4). Bilateral symmetry is usually noted, as is dominant inheritance. Degeneration of the deposit, with secondary fibrous infiltrate and visual loss, is reported in many kinships with this disorder; however, some families never have visual symptoms. A defect in a specific electrophysiologic test, the electro-oculogram, is pathognomonic for this disorder.

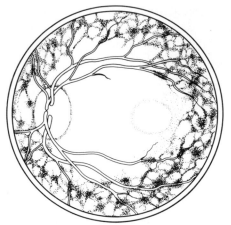

Figure 7-3. Retinitis pigmentosa. A bone-spicule pattern of paravascular pigmentation.

DEGENERATIONS OF THE CHOROID

Degenerations of the choroid are quite uncommon; the most frequently reported representative is choroideremia. This is an X-linked disorder of variable expressivity. The female carrier has diffuse pigment mottling of the ocular fundus. The young male with the disorder looks like the female carrier; however, in the first decade there is severe peripheral retinal and choroidal atrophy. This may progress to leave a residual central normally functioning

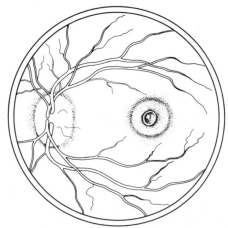

Figure 7-4. Vitelliform macular degeneration. A macular cyst of egg-yolk color.

island capable of seeing 20/20 while the patient is functionally and legally blind because of the extreme field loss.

DEVELOPMENTAL VARIATIONS

Coloboma

A coloboma is a commonly noted tissue defect. This defect is caused by inadequate closure of the fetal fissure of the eye. In embryologic development the optic vesicle invaginates on itself to produce a double-wall cup. This invagination occurs along the inferonasal portion of the optic vesicle. After invagination is complete, the resulting fissure is obliterated by fusion of the adjacent walls. When this closure is defective, a coloboma may develop. A coloboma appears as a depigmented and devascularized area, with the neurosensory retina in direct contact with the sclera. Unless additional problems develop, this defect remains an area of curiosity for which therapy is not indicated. However, retinal detachments associated with this disorder have a relatively poor prognosis and require specialized surgical therapy.[13]

Juvenile Retinoschisis

Juvenile retinoschisis is a sex-linked recessively inherited disorder. It is characterized by a splitting of the retina into two layers. The earliest clinical finding is a bullous cystlike lesion near the ocular equator in the inferotemporal quadrant.[8]

As the patient gets older this cyst will enlarge in every dimension. It may extend anteriorly, but it will rarely, if ever, contact the ora serrata. It may enlarge posteriorly until it is in contact with the optic nerve. Thinning of the inner layer is associated with many oval or round breaks in the schisis wall. Similar changes of the outer wall will permit the fluid within the schisis cavity to enter the subretinal space and will produce retinal detachment.

A perifoveal macular microschisis develops at some time in the life of each patient with this disorder. When this occurs, visual acuity may become reduced precipitously. In some families the perifoveal defects are noted before development of the midperipheral lesions. However, most reported patients maintain good vision until they are in their middle twenties.

There is no known therapy for this primary disorder. However, the associated retinal detachment, which can remove the residual vision of these patients, can be treated with routine retinal detachment surgery.

Myopic Degeneration

Myopic degeneration is another developmental defect of the eye. In approximately 10 percent of the American population there exists simple axial myopia, a condition in which the eyeball is longer than desirable for good focus. In a smaller percentage of patients the eye length is associated with pathologic changes. In the pediatric population these changes include vitreous separation and floaters, pigmentary crescents of the optic nerve, pigmentary degeneration of the macula, lattice degeneration of the peripheral retina, and retinal detachment.

The vitreous changes are most common. The vitreous can separate from the adjacent retina and can move within the eye. The motion of objects within the vitreous produces shadows on the retina. These particles are out of focus for the eye and appear as round or ameboid floaters.

A myopic crescent usually appears on the temporal margin of the optic nerve. It is frequently a depigmented crescent through which one can see choroid and sclera. This crescent may represent an abnormal enlargment of the eyeball. The inner ocular layer, the retina, cannot stretch enough to coat the outer layer, the choroid; the resulting gaplike defect is the crescent.

In some patients pathologic myopia is associated with abnormalities of the chorioretinal barrier layer. These produce subretinal hemorrhage, neovascularization, and pigment deposition. Frequently these changes result in a fibrotic scar and a central scotoma.

In the retinal periphery the tissues become thinner than normal. Inner retinal layer degeneration characterized by a latticework of retinal vessels is noted in many patients.

Approximately one-third of retinal detachment patients are noted to have a combination of vitreous separation and peripheral retinal lattice degeneration. However, less than 0.01 percent of all patients develop retinal detachments. Therefore pediatric patients with myopia, vitreous separation, and lattice degeneration are at great risk to develop this potentially blinding complication.

TRAUMA

Changes in the retina, vitreous, and choroid produced by trauma are common in the pediatric population. These are associated, in most cases, with concurrent damages to the adjacent structures that may produce equally significant problems.

Traumatic Retinopathy

Traumatic retinopathy has been described by several different authors. Historically, each different source of trauma was believed to produce an individual and distinct retinopathy. However, all are quite similar in that there is an abrupt shocklike increase in orbital intravascular pressure associated with transudation into the retina. This results in a clinical picture of exudates, hemorrhage, and retinal edema. In most cases this will resolve spontaneously without residual defects.

An exception to this pattern is sometimes noted in the commotio retinae associated with Berlin's edema. This is the variety produced by direct trauma to the eyeball. The sudden increase in vascular pressure is part of a generalized increase in intraocular pressure. Pressure necrosis of the neural tissue can occur that is not reversible. Nevertheless, the final visual outcome cannot be predicted until the edema resolves.

Retinal Dialysis

Retinal dialysis is a type of traumatic rhegmatogenous retinal detachment that is similar, in many ways, to that described earlier. Its distinguishing feature is that the break is not within the retina but at the border between the retina and the pars plana of the ciliary body.

This defect is produced in an indirect manner. The injury produces a reverberation within the vitreous gel; because of its consistency, the vitreous gel can move at a different rate than the retina. The vitreous is adherent to the retina in the border zone between the retina and pars plana, and the vitreous movement pulls and tears the retina at its edge. This can result in a technical surgical problem because the vitreous can come to lie beneath the retina and prevent the reapproximation of layers needed for surgical repair.

Penetrating Wounds

Many aspects of the therapy of penetrating ocular wounds are of importance. However, two features take precedence: closure of the wound and removal of the penetrating foreign body. The primary therapy must be closure of the ocular wound. Involuntary contraction of the extraocular muscles can cause rapid expulsion of the intraocular contents through the smallest opening. Frequently the penetrating foreign body will be at some distance from the lacerated wound edge. At such times it is important to close the laceration with microsurgical techniques and reappraise the location of the foreign body. It is common to find that the safest path for removal of the foreign body is through an incision at some distance from the entrance wound.

Localization and removal of the foreign body are of equal importance to wound closure. The techniques are difficult and often require the aid of specialists experienced in this field. The most frequently used procedures include orbital ultrasonography, computerized axial tomography, electromagnetic evaluation, and intravitreal manipulation during surgery.

An important complication of ocular trauma is sympathetic ophthalmia.

This is a rare disorder whose exact etiology is unknown. It is believed that rupture of the blood–eye barrier permits uveal antigens to stimulate an autoimmune response to ocular tissue. In such cases a penetrating injury to one eye can cause the loss of both eyes. Rapid enucleation of the traumatized eye may prevent this complication, but this has no effect on the disorder once it has started. Systemic cortiocosteroids can aid many patients in retaining useful vision in both eyes; however, in some cases careful medical therapy is unable to control the disorder.

INFECTIONS

Nematodes

Nematodes are a class of ocular parasites that are found in many parts of the world. In the United States, *Toxocara canis* is the most common member of this class of parasites.[14]

When the nematode invades other portions of the body, the condition is described as visceral larva migrans. It may be associated with eosinophilia, pneumonitis, and hepatosplenomegaly. However, when ocular involvement is noted, systemic manifestations are rare.

A wide spectrum of ocular findings is reported with this disorder. The most common feature is clouding of the vitreous by inflammatory cells. A large, single vitreous opacity from which radiate white fibrous bands is characteristic of this disorder. However, this parasite can appear as a tumor of the choroid, a nonrhegmatogenous retinal detachment, or a white mass obstructing the pupil.

Cutaneous and serologic tests for this parasite are not reliable. Therapy may be available if this disorder can be clinically distinguished from retinoblastoma. Direct mechanical removal or photocoagulation may cause exacerbation of the inflammation and loss of the eye. Indirect treatment with cycloplegics and steroids has permitted reduction of inflammation and the return of some vision. If vision is lost, retention of the eye may permit the patient to maintain a better cosmetic appearance than would be possible following enucleation.

Protozoa

Toxoplasmosis is a common cause of posterior ocular inflammation in children. Two forms of this disorder are believed to exist: a congenital variety and an acquired variety. Usually the congenital form has bilateral chorioretinitis, hepatosplenomegaly, hydrocephalus, and intracerebral calcifications. Unilateral chorioretinitis may be the only manifestation of the acquired disease.

The chorioretinal lesions appear as well-circumscribed punched-out areas in the retina and pigment epithelium. They tend to fluctuate in activity; this may be indicated by changes in the degree of vitreal clouding. Exacerbations may be associated with extension of the disorder to create a satellite lesion adjacent to the original chorioretinal scar. In addition to this clinical picture, a serum antibody test will help to confirm the diagnosis.

Therapy with sulfadiazine, pyrimethamine, and folinic acid has been of of benefit to most patients with this disorder.[15] Neither systemic steroid therapy nor photocoagulation therapy has been proved beneficial in a reproducible manner for such patients; however, individual case reports have attributed improvement to these modalities of treatment.

Viruses

The most common viral retinopathy in the pediatric population is congenital rubella. It may be associated with cataract and microphthalmia, or it may be present as a singular finding. On clinical examination the retina has a mottled appearance; areas of hyperpigmentation alternate with areas of depigmentation, giving a salt-and-pepper pattern.

Unless other disorders are present, this abnormality is stationary. When the retinopathy is the only manifestation, all of the ocular functions are in the normal range.

HEMOGLOBINOPATHIES

Disorders involving different hemoglobin molecules are of special interest. They may differ by a single amino acid. The most common hemoglobin is type A; less often, hemoglobins S, C, or others are identified. The presence of S hemoglobin permits deformation of the red blood cells and secondary circulatory disturbances. Patients who are homozygous for hemoglobin S have sickle cell disease and severe systemic manifestations. The heterozygous state can be sickle trait (SA), or it can be SC hemoglobin disease. Retinal findings may be present in all patients who have hemoglobin S, but because of the reduced systemic findings, ocular changes represent the major manifestations in heterozygous patients with SA or SC. The typical retinal lesion in a patient with SS is the "black sunburst." This is a round, darkly pigmented lesion up to 3 mm in diameter located in the midperiphery of the eye. The center of this lesion may represent an intraretinal arteriolar occlusion.

The typical retinal lesion in SC is the "sea fan." This represents retinal neovascularization that projects into the vitreous from the midperiphery of the eye. The neovascularization probably represents a response to incomplete retinal infarction. Nevertheless, the neovascularization is a potential cause of severe visual loss. The new vessels are more fragile than preexisting vessels, and they tend to rupture, producing vitreal hemorrhages. This can be a cause of intravitreal gliosis and tractional retinal detachments.[16]

METABOLIC DISORDERS

The most common metabolic disorder involving the retina is diabetes mellitus. Although the sequelae of diabetic retinopathy are the most common causes of blindness in the United States, this is rarely a pediatric problem. The available data indicate that the retinal complications are related to the duration of the disease. In general, the insulin-dependent juvenile-onset diabetic will have the disorder more than 15 years before retinal changes are demonstrable. A recent report from the Diabetic Retinopathy Study Group of the National Institutes of Health indicates that sight-preserving therapy is available for many patients.[17] The beneficial treatment consists of focal photocoagulation to destroy the developing neovascularization, as well as panretinal photocoagulation to destroy the tissues that may be stimuli to future neovascularization.

UVEITIS

The uvea consists of the major vascular portions of the eye. An inflammation of the uvea, uveitis, can be described in terms of the specific tissues involved. When the iris is involved the disorder is iritis; when the ciliary body is involved, cyclitis; when the choroid is involved, choroiditis; when all portions of the uvea are equally involved, panuveitis. Specific uveal inflammatory disorders associated with known etiologic agents are discussed in the appropriate sections. However, there are some general trends in uveal inflammation, and there are varieties of uveitis whose etiologies remain unknown. For this reason a separate discussion of these features follows.

In general endogenous uveitis can be divided into granulomatous and nongranulomatous varieties on the basis of cellular reactions. In an eye with granulomatous uveitis, clusters of cells can be found that contain polymorphonuclear leukocytes, lymphocytes, epithelioid cells, and an occasional giant cell. A nongranulomatous response is one in which the cell clusters are characterized by lymphocytes and plasma cells.

Granulomatous uveitis may be caused by bacterial, viral, mycotic, and parasitic agents. In some cases the etiology can be determined by tissue biopsy and culture. However, often the etiology remains unknown, and the biopsy technique may cause more damage to the eye than the primary disorder.

Granulomatous uveitis may originate as a slowly developing insidious cellular response. A vascular reaction that results in increasing protein in the aqueous fluid (the development of anterior chamber flare) may gradually develop. Clusters of inflammatory cells may be present within the uveal tissue, floating with the ocular media, or adherent to adjacent structures. These may adhere to the walls of the anterior chamber and may, in part, be related to the development of synechiae.

Nongranulomatous uveitis is usually associated with acute onset. There is marked congestion of the vascular tissues and photophobia. The vascular dilation is associated with an intense outpouring of protein into the aqueous (flare). The cellular response described above is associated with fine pinpoint deposits on the walls of the anterior chamber. No nodules are noted, but synechiae may develop in eyes with protein-containing exudates. The etiologic agent of nongranulomatous uveitis is rarely identified.

Table 7-1 describes the most common causes of uveitis. However, it must be emphasized that many uveitis cases have unknown etiology. The percentage of cases with unknown etiology varies in regard to which publication is cited; however, an average of 30 percent is frequently mentioned.

If the inciting agent cannot be identified and treated, a regimen that can minimize visual loss and reduce the inflammatory reaction is needed. Every medication that can be of value in this manner is associated with local and systemic complications; therefore, frequent repetitive examinations by an expert are required.

The therapeutic agents with the fewest side effects are the mydriatics. Their major function in uveitis is to reduce muscle spasm of the ciliary body and iris and reduce photophobia. The choice of mydriatic varies according to the severity of the disorder, the experience of the physician, and the reactivity of the patient. The local side effects of mydriatric agents include blurring of vision and loss of accommodation, acute glaucoma attacks in patients with congenital narrow angles, and contact dermatitis. The systemic effects include dryness and flushing of the skin, thirst, tachycardia, delirium, and confusion.

Corticosteroids can be used with great benefit; however, they must be used with extreme caution. Some agents that cause uveitis, such as the bacteria, fungi, and viruses, can be stimulated by cortiocosteroids. When applied topically, corticosterioids have been reported to produce pathologic rises in intraocular pressure in 30 percent of patients maintained on this drug for more than 3 weeks. Topical, subconjunctival, and systemic corticosteroids have been associated with increased incidences of posterior subcapsular cataracts. In some series as many as 80 percent of patients who have had uveitis treated with corticosteroids for more than 1 year have developed some cataractous

Table 7–1
Common Causes of Uveitis

Histoplasmosis
Toxoplasmosis
Sarcoidosis
Syphilis
Toxocara canis
Virus (herpes simplex, herpes zoster, others)
Ankylosing spondylitis
Tuberculosis
Phacoanaphylactic response
Trauma
Brucellosis
Ulcerative colitis
Coccidioidomycosis
Behçet's syndrome
Sympathetic ophthalmia
Vogt-Koyanagi-Harada syndrome
Immune complex disorders

changes. For these many reasons it is strongly recommended that an ophthalmologist supervise this form of therapy.

ENUCLEATION

It is uncommon to perform enucleation in a pediatric patient. However, the disorders of the retina, vitreous, and choroid are the pediatric ocular problems that most often result in enucleation. If the blind eye is not growing at a normal rate, orbital and facial growth is somewhat reduced; if the eye is removed, the stimulus for growth is less. In a pediatric patient, a prosthesis will need to be revised continually and may require frequent reoperations. In general, an ophthalmic plastic surgeon will be needed to balance the development of both sides of the patient's face in a manner that will result in the best cosmetic appearance.[18]

REFERENCES

1.   Havener WA: Ocular Pharmacology. St Louis, CV Mosby, 1970
2.   Fraunfelder FT, Scafidi AF: Possible adverse effects from topical ocular 10% phenylephrine. Am J Ophthalmol 85:447, 1978

3. James LS, Lanman JT (eds): History of oxygen therapy and retrolental fibrop-
    lasia. Pediatrics (Suppl) 57:1, 1976
4. Patz A: Retrolental fibroplasia. Surv Ophthalmol 14:1, 1969
5. Reese AB: Persistent hyperplastic primary vitreous. Am J Ophthalmol 42:1,
    1956
6. Wise GN, Dollery CT, Henkind P: The Retinal Circulation. New York, Harper
    & Row, 1971, p 256
7. Ellsworth RM: Retinoblastoma, diseases of the retina, in Duane TD (ed): Clini-
    cal Ophthalmology, vol 3. Hagerstown, Md, Harper & Row, 1976
8. Yanoff M, Rahn EK, Zimmerman LE: Histopathology of juvenile retinoschisis.
    Arch Ophthalmol 79:49, 1968
9. Tasman W: Retinal Diseases in Children. New York, Harper & Row, 1971
10. Schenk L, Friedlander J, Valenti L, Adachi M, Amsterdam O, Volk BW: Pre-
    natal diagnosis in Tay-Sachs disease. Lancet 1:582, 1970
11. Cogan DG: Heredodegenerations of the retina, in Lawton Smith J (ed): Neuro-
    ophthalmology, vol 2. St Louis, CV Mosby, 1965, p 44
12. Krill AE: Retinitis Pigmentosa. A Review. Sight Sav Rev 42:21, 1972
13. Jesberg DO, Schepens CL: Retinal detachment associated with coloboma of the
    choroid. Arch Ophthalmol 65:163, 1960
14. Wilder HC: Nematode endophthalmitis. Trans Am Acad Ophthalmol Otolaryn
    gol. 1950, p 99
15. O'Connor GR: Manifestations and management of ocular toxoplasmosis. Bull
    NY Acad Med 50:192, 1974
16. Goldberg MF: Classification and pathogenesis or proliferative sickle retinopathy.
    Am J Ophthalmol 71:646, 1971
17. Diabetic Retinopathy Study Research Group: Preliminary report on effects of
    photocoagulation therapy. Am J Ophthalmol 81:383, 1976
18. Kennedy RE: The effect of early enucleation on the orbit. Am J Ophthalmol
    60:277, 1965

Ian H. Porter, M.D.

8
Principles and Examples in Ophthalmic Genetics

INTRODUCTION

Deoxyribonucleic acid (DNA) is the hereditary material. It participates in two processes: one is replication, its genetic function; the other is transcription, its biochemical function. That strip of DNA that carries the code for the sequence of amino acids in a polypeptide chain is a gene, the unit of heredity. There probably are about 50,000 structural genes in man, of which only about 1100 autosomal genes and 100 genes in the X chromosome have been identified on the basis of characteristic patterns of inheritance.

Linkage

Particular genes are situated at specific sites, or loci, in chromosomes. There are 46 chromosomes: 22 homologous pairs and 2 sex chromosomes, an X and a Y. In each pair of chromosomes one member is paternal and one is maternal in origin. As chromosomes exist in pairs, so also must genes; as the members of homologous chromosome pairs segregate, or separate, during the formation of gametes, so also must genes. On the other hand, when two genes are located in different chromosomes, the two characters they control will appear in the next generation either together or apart, depending on chance alone. They assort independently.

If two genes are in the same chromosome pair and are fairly close to each other, they will tend to be inherited together. They will not assort independently, and they are said to be linked. Occasionally, however, crossing-over

143

will occur between the genes at meiosis, and the two characters will part in some children. When a pair of genes is in the same chromsome, the chance that crossing-over will happen between them is greater the farther apart they are. If the two loci are close together, there is little room for a crossover to occur. The number of crossovers, therefore, is the measure of the distance between the genes.

On the basis of family and somatic cell hybridization studies, the gene map of human chromosomes now shows assignment of at least one structural gene locus to all 22 autosomes plus the X and Y chromosomes. More than 20 loci have been assigned to chromosome 1, including the Rh locus. The locus for the ABO blood groups is in chromosome 9, and the locus for the major histocompatibility complex is in chromosome 6. Of more than 100 loci assigned to the X chromosome, some information on their relative positions is available for at least 16 (Fig. 8-1). The Y chromosome contains genes that determine the normal development of testes and the H-Y histocompatibility antigens.

Genes with similar functions often are clustered in the same chromosome. For example, the genes for three enzymes involved in the Embden-Meyerhof pathway, glyceraldehyde-3-phosphate dehydrogenase (GAPD), triophosphate isomerase (TPI), and lactic dehydrogenase B (LDHв) are in chromosome 12. Linkage probably persists between loci that determine simi-

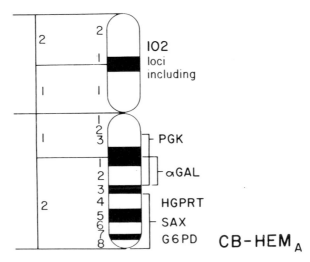

Figure 8-1.   Diagrammatic synopsis of gene map of human X chromosome. Banding pattern and numbering are those given in the 1975 supplement of the report of the Paris Conference (see Fig. 8-11).

lar proteins because they arose by gene duplication, as in the case, for example, with the loci for the different clusters of immunoglobulin genes, the genes for β-δ-γ polypeptide chains of hemoglobin, and the components of HLA.

Association

Association is the concurrence of two characters more often than would be expected by chance. It is different from linkage, in which the concurrence of two traits is not greater than expected by chance. Linkage is a phenomenon occurring between two genes in the same chromosome, whereas association may occur between a character controlled by a single gene and one controlled by many. Also, linkage has no etiologic significance, being merely an anatomic fact, whereas association may be causal.

The best-known example of association is that between blood groups and diseases of the upper gastrointestinal tract. The incidence of cancer of the stomach, pernicious anemia, and salivary gland tumors is significantly higher in people with blood group A than in people with group O. Similarly, there is an association between peptic ulcer and blood group O. The most recent and most interesting examples of association are those betweeen HLA antigens and ankylosing spondylitis, Reiter's syndrome, and psoriatic arthritis.

These associations vary in both strength and specificity. For example, individuals with the B27 antigen have nearly a 100-fold greater risk of developing ankylosing spondylitis, but only an eight-fold greater risk of developing psoriatic arthritis, than those without the B27 antigen.

There are three explanations for these populations' associations. First, the association may be an artifact of sampling from a heterogeneous population that contains a subgroup in which both the antigen and the disease exist at frequencies higher than in the remainder of the population. Such stratification is common in ethnically mixed populations. Second, the disease susceptibility may be a direct result of the presence of the particular HLA antigen. In the mouse, for example, certain H-2 antigens appear to facilitate viral infection or modify immunologic response to such infections. Third, linkage disequilibrium may exist between the alleles for the antigen(s) studied and the alleles at nearby loci that actually control susceptibility to the disease. Linkage disequilibrium is a tendency in a population for some alleles at closely linked loci to occur together in the same chromosome more often than expected by chance.

Mutation

DNA has two characteristics: it is remarkably stable, and it replicates identically. If this were not true, the orderly development of an individual and the stability of the species would not be possible. On the other hand, if we were all identical, then the question of inheritance might never have arisen, because it is the difference that provides us with the observational units in genetics. One of the causes of individual variation is mutation. A mutation of any nucleotide will result in one of the amino acids making up a polypeptide being substituted for another. As a result, the polypeptide will be altered. Some of these changes may not have much effect, some may lead to only slight variation, and others may cause disease or may even be lethal. Medical genetics is the study of those differences in the genotype that under certain conditions may lead to disease and are merely selective examples of all the differences that make each one of us unique (with, perhaps, the exception of identical twins).

Allelism

If a man with an identical gene, say A, at a given locus of the homologous chromosome, i.e., with an AA genotype, married a woman with the same gene at both loci, i.e., also with an AA genotype, then only gametes with the A gene, and consequently only children with the AA genotype, can result. If, on the other hand, A exists in another form (an allele, say a) and the genotype of the father is AA and the genotype of the mother is Aa, then the father will produce only A gametes, but half the mother's gametes will be A and half will be a. The possible genotypes of the children will then be

$$AA \times Aa = AA:AA:Aa:Aa$$

So half the children will have the genotype AA and half the children will have the genotype Aa. If both parents have the genotype Aa, the one-fourth of the children will have the genotype AA or aa, and half the children will have the genotype Aa:

$$Aa \times Aa = AA:Aa:aA:aa$$

When a gene exists in alternate forms in a population (A and a) there are three possible genotypes, and when a gene has three alleles (A, a, and a') there are six possible genotypes:

$$AA, Aa, Aa', aa, aa', and a' a'$$

In other words, the more allelic forms in which the gene exists in a population, the larger is the number of possible genotypes.

Many alleles may be generated from a single gene by separate mutational events. For example, from a gene containing a sequence of 900 DNA nucleotide bases and coding for a polypeptide of 300 amino acids, 2700 alleles, each differing from the original by only a single base change, may be formed by separate mutations, since each of the 900 bases may be altered to one of the three others in different mutational events. Some 20–25 percent of all mutations of this type, however, will be synonymous. That is to say, they will result in no alteration in amino acid structure of the polypeptide, because it will simply involve a change of a particular codon to another specifying the same amino acid. In about 4 percent of cases, mutation will cause an alteration of a base triplet coding for an amino acid to a nonsence triplet which results in chain termination and leads to considerable disruption of protein structure and loss of functional activity.

It turns out that if we investigate any protein or enzyme, there usually are one or two common variants in the population (frequencies greater than 1:1000), and then there are usually a number of rare ones (frequencies less than 1:10,000). Any individual may be heterozygous at about 16 percent of all gene loci. If there are 50,000 structural genes, one would expect that in any single person there may be about 8000 loci at which there are two different alleles resulting in the synthesis of structurally distinct forms of a particular polypeptide. The 50,000 structural genes include those that determine the basic structure of all structural proteins, all proteins of special function, such as hemoglobins and immunoglobulins, the amino acid structure of many enzymes involved in processing proteins, such as procollagen peptidase and proline and lysine hydroxylases necessary for formation of collagen fibers, and, of course, those involved in intermediary metabolism.

Inborn Errors of Metabolism

A mutation, then, is a simple base substitution of DNA leading to a single amino acid substitution in a polypeptide. If it so alters the properties of an enzyme involved in intermediary metabolism that it leads to a metabolic block, we have an inborn error of metabolism, which has the following characteristics (Fig. 8-2): (1) high serum levels of the substrate proximal to the metabolic block; (2) a serum deficiency of the product distal to the block; (3) excess excretion in the urine of the substrate; (4 and 5) secondary metabolic effects. Thus an inborn error of metabolism is a disease with characteristic clinical, pathologic, and biochemical abnormalities attributable to an alteration in the activity of a specific enzyme that, in turn, is due to the presence of a particular abnormal gene.

Phenylketonuria.   Phenylketonuria (PKU) is the model inborn error of metabolism. The enzyme defect has been demonstrated, the mode of inheritance has been determined, and treatment is available.

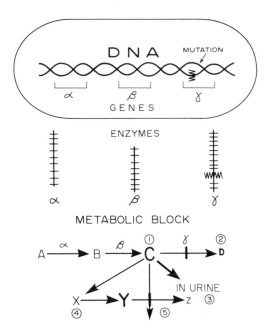

Figure 8-2.   Schematic representation of a mutation leading to a
single amino acid substitution producing a metabolic block.

PKU is a disorder of amino acid metabolism. The enzyme phenylalanine
hydroxylase, which normally converts phenylalanine to tyrosine, is defective,
which results in high levels of serum phenylalanine, low levels of serum
tyrosine, and excretion of phenylpyruvic acid and other abnormal metabolites
in the urine. It is inherited as a recessive condition, and the incidence is
approximately 1 in 10,000 births. The characteristic features of PKU are
severe mental retardation and other neurologoic abnormalities. However,
children with PKU are normal at birth because the maternal enzyme protects
them during prenatal life; they become retarded only when fed phenylalanine.
    The consequences of the enzymatic block can be circumvented by giving
a diet low in phenylalanine. The results are best when the diagnosis is made
soon after birth and treatment is begun promptly and is continued for an
as-yet-undetermined time, but probably longer than the customary 4–5 years.
    Because genes control metabolic pathways, and because mutations occur
constantly and randomly (that is to say, all parts of the genetic material are
equally susceptible), we might expect eventually to discover an increasing
number of inborn errors of metabolism. We would expect to discover not only

an inborn error of metabolism involving every step in every metabolic pathway, i.e., mutations of different genes, but also, as we have seen, many variants of each enzyme, i.e., mutations of the same gene (alleles). Thus, for example, inborn errors of metabolism are known for each step of the pentose phosphate shunt, the first step of which is catalyzed by glucose-6-phosphate dehydrogenase (G-6-PD). There are 80 known variants of G-6-PD that can be attributed to different mutant alleles at a single locus in the X chromosome. A few of these variants are common in certain populations and give rise to hemolytic disease when people who have them are exposed to certain drugs, but most of them are rare and seem to have no adverse effects. At the present rate of discovery, there will be about 12,000 inborn errors of metabolism in the year 2009—the centenary of the publication of Sir Archibald Garrod's "Inborn Errors of Metabolism."

MODES OF INHERITANCE

Autosomal Recessive Inheritance

There are about 500 known recessive disorders, and most of the inborn errors of metabolism are inherited as recessive (X-linked) conditions. Patients with the typical clinical and metabolic features of these conditions are homozygotes for the particular gene, whereas the parents are heterozygotes.

The effect of a gene that is recognizable only in the homozygous state is recessive. The homozygous state can occur only if both parents possess the gene with the abnormal effect. Thus recessive defects are inherited from both parents, who apparently are normal, but each carries the gene for the trait in one of the relevant pair of chromosomes.

In a marriage between heterozygotes, both parents produce normal and abnormal gametes in equal proportions. There are four possibilities:

Maternal Gametes

		A	a
Paternal Gametes	A	AA	Aa
	a	Aa	aa

$$AA—2Aa—aa$$

Because the condition is recessive, we have three apparently normal children and one affected child. With the recessive condition, the tendency is for certain defects to appear in more than one member of the sibship born to apparently normal parents. Often the parents are related, because the probability that a rare gene is present in both parents is greater if they have common ancestry and, thus, common genes. A gene with a recessive effect may be handed down through many generations of heterozygotes, and its existence will, of course, be quite unsuspected. Only when a heterozygote marries another heterozygote can the homozygote appear.

In summary, then, the criteria for recognizing autosomal recessive inheritance are (Figs. 8-3 and 8.4):

1. Patients are homozygotes.
2. Patients are the children of apparently normal parents.
3. Often, more than one child in the sibship is affected. On the average, one-quarter of the sibs of the proband are affected. Boys are affected as often as girls.
4. Affected people who marry normal people have apparently normal children.
5. In rare recessive conditions, there is an undue proportion of related marriages among the parents of probands. Indeed, the rarer the defect, the higher the proportion of consanguineous marriages.

CONSANGUINITY

Consanguinity occurs in less than 1 percent of marriages in most Western countries, but there are isolated areas and societies where the consanguinity rate is as high as 25 percent. As one might expect, it is more common in small, isolated rural populations than in large cities.

The relative risk of a consanguineous marriage refers to the chance that such a marriage will produce an affected child, as compared with the chance that a random marriage will produce a similarly affected child. It is about the same as the percentage of first-cousin marriages among parents of affected children. Thus, a cousin marriage is approximately 10 times more likely to produce a child with PKU than a random marriage, since the percentage of consanguinity among the parents of children with the disease is about 10 percent.

Closely consanguineous marriages are a high-risk group for rare recessive conditions, and certain marriages have, at least in part, for genetic reasons, been outlawed as a public health measure.

Consider a group of 16 families, each with 2 children and with all parents heterozygotes for a rare gene with a recessive effect (Figure 8-5). As the chance of having an affected child is 1 in 4, the chances are that 4 of the 16 first-born children will be affected. The chance of having two affected children is 1 in 16 ($\frac{1}{4} \times \frac{1}{4}$), since the chance of having a second affected child is

AUTOSOMAL RECESSIVE INHERITANCE

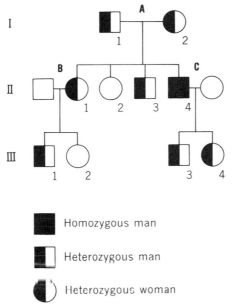

Figure 8-3. Pedigree demonstrating the results of marriages (A) between two carriers (heterozygotes) for a recessive condition (B) between a normal man and a heterozygous woman, and (C) between a homozygous man and a normal woman (see Fig. 8-4).

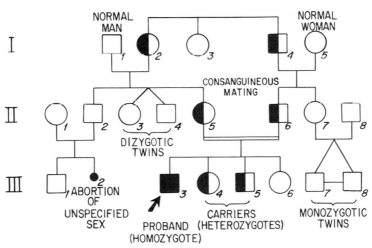

Figure 8-4. Conventional symbols used in drawing pedigrees.

not influenced by whether or not the first is affected. But nine of the families will have no affected children. So, of the 16 families there will be six families with one affected child, one family with two affected children, and nine families with no affected children. There are, in other words, large numbers of couples in the population who are at risk of having affected children, but who do not, in fact, have them. Until recently, such couples become known only after they had had affected children. One reason for screening is to detect couples at risk before they have children.

SCREENING

There are certain groups of people who are known to be at risk for specific disorders that lend themselves to screening before these people have affected children. The aim is to detect carriers (heterozygotes) in such groups and hence identify couples at risk who may have affected offspring, e.g., Tay-Sachs disease in Ashkenazi Jews, sickle cell disease in blacks, and thalassemia in people of Mediterranean origin.

Tay-Sachs disease.   Tay-Sachs disease is an ideal disorder for screening for the following reasons: (1) it is mainly confined to a defined population; (2) there is a simple, reliable, automated, and relatively inexpensive test for detecting the carrier state; (3) the disorder can be diagnosed prenatally. Because about 1 in 30 Ashkenazi Jews of central and eastern European ancestry are carriers, the chance of two carriers marrying each other is $1/30 \times 1/30 = 1/900$. Because it is a recessive condition, the chance of them having an affected child is $1/900 \times 1/4 = 1/3600$.

In contrast, the disorder occurs rarely in all other populations, including Sephardic Jews, who have a carrier rate of about 1 in 100; thus their chance of having an affected child is $1/100 \times 1/100 \times 1/4 = 40,000$.

Tay-Sachs disease is one of the sphingolipidoses, in which DM_2 ganglioside accumulates in neuronal cells. Affected children, lack hexosaminidase A (Hex A) activity, and carriers have reduced enzyme activity.

The symptoms of Tay-Sachs disease start at about the age of 6 months, when a previously normally developing child starts to regress. There is apathy, loss of previously acquired function, and failure of vision, with development of the well-known cherry-red spot of the fundi. Later, seizures, hyperacusis, and increasing spasticity occur, leading to death, usually before the age of 2 years.

Couples who are both carriers should be counseled and should have their reproductive alternatives explained. They must be informed that they have a 25 percent chance of having an affected or a normal child and a 50 percent

SECOND CHILD

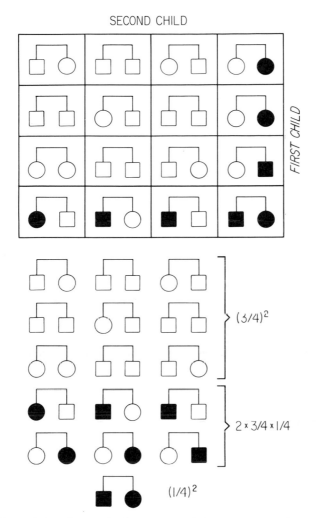

Figure 8-5. Group of 16 families with 2 children in which all parents are heterozygous for a recessive condition. Solid symbols indicate affected children. Note that only 7 of the 16 families will be ascertained when the families are found because of at least one affected child.

chance of having a child who is a carrier like themselves. It is now possible to monitor pregnancies and measure the activity of Hex A in cells obtained from amniotic fluid.

If all Ashkenazi Jews of childbearing age in America were screened for the Tay-Sachs gene, and if all the couples were able to have 2 chidlren (none with Tay-Sachs disease), the overall effect would be a relative increase in the gene frequency of 0.09 percent per 25-year generation. Therefore, it would take thousands of years for the frequency of heterozygotes for Tay-Sachs disease to change significantly. Thus, from a public health point of view, we need not be greatly concerned.

PKU.   Another reason for screening is to detect patients (homozygotes) for the purpose of treatment. Screening for this purpose was begun in the United States in 1963 for PKU, and 43 states now have laws requiring or recommending PKU screening in newborns. These programs are undertaken with the following assumptions: (1) PKU can be detected in the newborn; (2) if untreated, PKU results in severe mental retardation; (3) restriction of phenylalanine intake started soon after birth prevents the development of mental retardation in infants with PKU.

Dietary restriction was the first successful form of treatment in patients with inborn errors of metabolism when the value of a low-phenylalanine diet to limit the accumulation of toxic substrate in patients with PKU was demonstrated in 1953. Subsequent experience also has proved this mode of treatment effective for patients with other inborn errors of metabolism whose pathogeneses are characterized by toxic substrate accumulation, e.g., galactosemia, hereditary fructose intolerance, lactose intolerance, and tyrosinemia.

The success of the PKU programs and advances in ability to screen for and confirm the diagnoses of other inborn errors of metabolism have led to expansion of many screening programs. Thus several states now have one or more of the following added to their original screening programs: galactosemia, maple syrup urine disease, homocystinuria, tyrosinosis, histidinemia, and other renal transport disorders.

The incidence of PKU would be increased only about 20 percent in 100 generations if children with PKU were to live to become normal reproductive adults; so one should not be unduly alarmed by the long-term public health effects of this type of screening program either.

Note that an essential aspect of screening for carriers or heterozygotes for the purpose of detecting couples at risk is availability of prenatal diagnosis, and an essential aspect of screening for patients or homozygotes is availability of treatment.

There are now about 80 inborn errors of metabolism that can be detected prenatally, but most of them are so rare that screening for them is not practicable.

Autosomal Dominant Inheritance

There are about 600 known dominant conditions. Dominant conditions tend to have a later stage of onset and to be less severe than recessive conditions; they are often morphologic and are not easily explained in biochemical terms. The effect of a gene that is recognized in the homozygous and heterozygous states is dominant. We usually do not come across homozygotes for dominant conditions because they can occur only as a result of a marriage between two heterozygotes, and dominant conditions are so rare that a marriage between heterozygotes seldom occurs. Consider, for example, a dominant condition with an incidence of 1 in 5000. The homozygote for this gene would be expected to occur once in 25 million people. So the chance of affected heterozygotes marrying similarly affected heterozygotes is remote, to say the least.

The chance of a child of an affected heterozygote and a normal parent being affected is 50 percent because the affected parent may, with equal likelihood, give either the gene with the normal effect or the mutant gene to any one of the children. Since the gene is carried in one of the autosomes, sons and daughters are equally likely to be affected.

In summary, then, the criteria for recognizing autosomal dominant inheritance are(Fig. 8–6) the following:

1. Patients are heterozygotes.
2. Patients have one affected parent (unless the gene with the abnormal effect was the result of a new mutation).
3. Boys and girls are equally likely to be affected.
4. Normal family members do not transmit the abnormality to their children unless the effect of the gene is subclinical.

PENETRANCE

The severity of dominant conditions varies considerably. This is exemplified by Marfan's syndrome, a condition characterized by upwardly dislocated lenses, excessive length of the limbs, and dissecting and/or diffuse aneurysm of the ascending aorta. Some patients have all three of these major clinical manifestations; others have only a few; in still others the signs are so mild that they cannot be detected clinically.

The people who possess but do not express the effect of the gene product may nevertheless transmit the abnormality to their children. Cases of forme fruste, or of incomplete penetrance, are analogous to the subclinical signs of infectious diseases. The gene with a dominant effect is fully penetrant when the character it controls can always be detected in homozygotes. *Penetrance is the frequency with which effect is shown in a population.* Lack of penetrance is one reason for skipped generations, unexpected pedigree patterns, and unusual genetic ratios.

AUTOSOMAL DOMINANT INHERITANCE

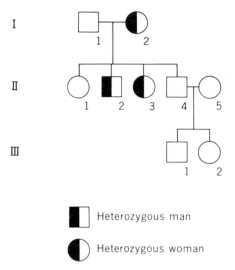

Figure 8-6. Pedigree demonstrating the results of a marriage between a normal man and an affected (heterozygous) woman for a
dominant condition.

EXPRESSIVITY

Some patients with Marfan's syndrome are severely affected and have all
three major anomalies, whereas others are mildly affected and have only
dislocated lenses. In genetic jargon, severity is referred to as expressivity.
Expressivity is the degree to which the effects are shown in an individual.

PLEIOTROPY

The primary function of a gene is the synthesis of a polypeptide chain.
From this primary function, however, many different consequences may result. Multiple phenotypic effects produced by a single gene are called pleiotropic effects. For example, in Marfan's syndrome the pleiotropic effects
(ocular, skeletal, and cardiovascular) may have a common basis, a defect in
the elastic fibers of connective tissue. By contrast, in the Laurence-Moon-
Bardet-Biedl syndrome (mental retardation, obesity, hypogonadism, polydac-
tyly, deafness, and retinitis pigmentosa) there is no obvious common basis for
the assortment of abnormalities. There are many examples in the literature of
misinterpretation of the different aspects of hereditary syndromes in terms of
linkage rather than pleiotropy. The association of two or more traits in members of a family usually does not suggest linkage; it is much more likely to be

due to pleiotropic effects of a single gene. As an example, the syndrome of hereditary juvenile glaucoma and slate-blue eye color was at first described as an example of linkage of glaucoma and eye color genes. Were this so, one would expect that the two traits would remain together for two or three generations and then become separated by crossing over in some individual, thus establishing two lines, one with glaucoma but not with the characteristic eye color, and the other with slate-blue eyes but without glaucoma. From then on, the two traits would remain independent in those branches of the family. If, as we now know is the case, a single gene is responsible for both traits, they will always appear in the same individual; even if one trait is not expressed in a certain family member, it will nevertheless reappear in that member's descendants. The eye color and the glaucoma result from a developmental defect of the mesenchyme of the anterior chamber during embryonic life.

HETEROGENEITY

Heterogeneity is, in a sense, the opposite of pleiotropy: several genes, one effect. Thus when a genetic condition is examined closely, heterogeneity is usually discovered. That which first appeared to be a single clinical phenotypic entity is often found to be several clinically similar but genetically and biochemically distinct disorders. Genetic heterogeneity is of special interest and importance in the diagnosis of hereditary diseases. Similar phenotypes can be produced by the following means:

1 Mutations of different nucleotides in the same gene, exemplified by the hemoglobinopathies. Thus, for example, there are many different abnormal hemoglobins produced by mutations of the gene controlling the beta chain.

2. Mutations of different genes (genocopies), which can be detected by.

   A. Genetic observations. For example, Marfan's syndrome and homocystinuria are clinically quite similar, but the former is inherited as a dominant condition, whereas the latter is inherited as a recessive condition (Table 8–1). Similarly, there are dominant, recessive, and X-linked forms of retinitis pigmentosa (Table 8–2).

   B. Linkage relationships. An example is the deutan colorblindness gene that is quite close to the hemophilia A gene but is a long way from the hemophilia B (Christmas disease) gene in the X chromosome.

   C. Biochemical methods. Among the mucopolysaccharidoses (Table 8–3), the Hunter factor (a protein) will correct the defect in cultured fibroblasts from a patient with the Hunter syndrome without affecting normal cells or cells derived from patients with other types of mucopolysaccharidoses by accelerating mucopolysaccharide degradation.

3. Environmental agents (phenocopies). For example, the recessive condition of microcephaly and chorioretinopathy may be simulated by toxoplasmosis.

If neither of the parents of a person with a dominant condition shows the abnormality, then a new mutation may have occurred in one parent's gametes. Indeed, considerable proportions of all severe dominant anomalies are due to new mutations. In this situation one will, of course, not expect to find 50 percent of the siblings affected. As the mutations occur in only one gamete or one of the parents, only the child resulting from the fertilization of that gamete by a normal one will be affected. However, the children of the affected person will have a 50 percent chance of being affected.

MUTATION RATE

The frequency with which genes mutate spontaneously (the mutation rate) is of roughly the same order of magnitude in organisms as different as bacteria, *Drosophila,* and man. At each locus in each generation the mutation takes place about once in every half million people. But the mutation rate is usually expressed as the frequency of mutation per locus per gamete per generation. Since every person has two genes per locus, the mutation rate per gene corresponds to half the frequency of the newly occurring cases in the population. As each gene is present only once in the gamete, the mutation rate is the same as the number of mutations per gamete.

Table 8–1
Comparison of Homocystinuria and Marfan's Syndrome

	Homocystinuria	Marfan's Syndrome
Mode of inheritance	Recessive	Dominant
Skeletal abnormalities	Osteoporosis, fractures, occasional arachnodactyly	Arachnodacyly and loose-jointedness more striking
Pectus excavatum or carinatum	Frequent	Frequent
Ectopia lentis	Downward	Upward
Vascular disease	Dilatation with thrombosis in medium-size arteries and veins	Dilatation and/or dissection of aorta
Skin	Malar flush, livido reticularis	Striae distensae
Mental retardation	Frequent	Absent

Table 8–2
Examples of Inherited Ophthalmic Conditions

Dominant	Recessive	X-linked
Aniridia	Anophthalmia, complete	Cataracts
Anophthalmia and	Cataracts	Color blindness
microphthalmia	Coloboma of macula and	Leber's optic atrophy
Blepharochalasis and	skeletal anomalies	Macular dystrophy
double lip	Color blindness, total	Megalocornea
Blepharophimosis,	Corneal dystrophies	Microphthalmia and
epicanthus, inversus,	Cryptophthalmos and	mental deficiency
and ptosis	associated anomalies	Night blindness and
Cataracts	Cyclopia	myopia
Coloboma of iris	Ectopia lentis and ectopia	Nystagmus
Coloboma of macula	of pupil	Retinal detachment
Corneal dystropies	Glaucoma	Retinitis pigmentosa
Distichiasis	Glaucoma, juvenile	
Duane retraction syndrome	Macular degeneration,	
Ectopia lentis	juvenile	
Epicanthus	Microphthalmia	
Glaucoma, congenital	Night blindness and	
Glaucoma, juvenile	myopia	
Macular degeneration	Oguchi disease	
Microphthalmia and	Optic atrophy, congenital	
coloboma	Retinitis pigmentosa	
Microphthalmia and		
cataract		
Myopia		
Night blindness and myopia		
Nystagmus		
Optic atrophies		
Ptosis		
Retinal aplasia		
Retinal cone degeneration		
Retinal detachment		
Retinitis pigmentosa		
Retinoblastoma		
Rieger's syndrome		

An example of how to estimate a mutation rate for a dominant condition is the following: Of 1,054,985 births, 49 children with retinoblastoma were found with normal parents; therefore they represented cases of new mutations in one or the other of the two gametes received from the parents. So the mutation rate is $49/1,054,985 = 2.3 \times 10^{-5}$.

Some cases of retinoblastoma are not hereditary but sporadic, they result from two somatic mutational events in one cell. Risk estimates in families

Table 8-3

Mucopolysaccharidoses

MPS Type		Genetics*	Systemic Features		Ocular Features	
			Skeletal Dysplasia	*Mental Retardation*	*Corneal Clouding*	*Retinal Pigmentary Degeneration*
I-H:	Hurler	R ⎤ allelic	+++	+++	+++	+
I-S:	Scheie (formerly MPS-V)	R ⎦	+	±	+++	+
II:	Hunter	X ⎤ allelic				
	A: severe phenotype		+++	+++	–	+
	B: mild phenotype	X ⎦	++	±	+	+
III:	Sanfilippo	R ⎤ nonallelic				
	A: sulfatase-deficient		±	+++	–	+
	B: glucosaminidase-deficient	R ⎦	±	+++	–	+
IV:	Morquio	R	+++	±	++	–
V:	Vacant; now MPS-I-S					
VI:	Maroteaux-Lamy	R ⎤ allelic				
	A: severe phenotype		+++	–	++	–
	B: mild phenotype	R ⎦	+	–	++	–

*R = autosomal recessive; X = X-linked recessive.

with retinoblastoma are as follows: (1) two or more cases in a family: 50 percent; (2) sporadic unilateral case: 5 percent for sibs and offspring; (3) sporadic bilateral case: 10 percent for sibs and 40 percent for offspring. The locus of retinoblastoma is in the long arm of chromosome 13 (see Table 8–11).

X-linked Inheritance

There are about 100 known X-linked conditions. The rules of dominance and recessivity also apply to sex-linked or, better, X-linked inheritance. Since the homologous genes exist only in women who have two X chromosomes, only in them do X-linked genes have a dominant or recessive effect like autosomal genes. The problem of dominance or recessivity does not arise in men, who have only one X chromosome and therefore lack paired X-borne genes. If a man carries a gene with an abnormal effect in his X chromosome, he is abnormal. If he carries a gene with a normal effect in his X chromosome, he is normal. Because a boy does not receive his father's X chromosome, the characteristic finding in X-linkage is absence of male-to-male transmission

One can distinguish X-linked conditions from autosomal dominant conditions limited to men by assuring (1) that affected men married to normal women never have affected boys, (2) that the relevant locus and an X-linked marker locus are linked, and (3) that the incidence in women with XO Turner's syndrome is about the same as in men. One can exclude autosomal dominant conditions limited to women, but only by demonstrating linkage with an established X-linked trait. In summary, then, the criteria for recognizing X-linked inheritance are (Fig. 8–7) the following:

1. Affected boys are hemizygous.
2. Fifty percent of daughters are carriers.
3. Fifty percent of sons are affected.
4. Affected fathers do not have affected sons.
5. All daughters of affected fathers are carriers.

Multifactorial Inheritance

Many common diseases clearly are not inherited in a simple mendelian manner. There may be an underlying genetic predisposition that is reflected in a relatively higher concordance rate among monozygotic twins than among dizygotic twins and a higher frequency among relatives of patients than in the general population. So far, these congenital defects have neither been identified nor associated with single metabolic defects, nor with detectable chromosomal anomalies. Rather, they are determined by polygenic inheritance, i.e., by the interaction of alleles at a number of different loci, each contributing a small effect. Environmental factors also play a significant role in the determination of polygenic disorders of multifactorial etiology. The evidence for polygenic inheritance is based on data concerning incidence in the general population and data concerning the familial recurrence of particular malformations.

Thus, for example, in anencephaly and spina bifida, if 2 children in a family are already affected, the incidence in subsequent children is twice that in families where only 1 child was previously affected. Empirical data are also available for cleft lip and palate, atrial septal defect, congenital pyloric stenosis, and clubfoot. Glaucoma and strabismus are ophthalmic conditions that may be multifactorially inherited. In general, the recurrence risk for an affected first-degree relative of a single affected person is low (about 5 percent) and reflects the interaction of multiple genetic and environmental factors (Table 8–4).

In conditions determined by major mutant genes, the risk of recurrence is constant, regardless of whether the parents have had one or more affected children; but in polygenic conditions the risk of recurrence varies, since it is not a matter of presence or absence of a gene with an abnormal effect but of the family's average component of risk. In fact, the more members of the family affected and the more severe the malformation in the proband, the

X-LINKED RECESSIVE INHERITANCE

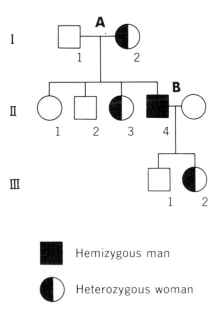

Figure 8-7.   Pedigree demonstrating the results of a marriage between (A) a normal man and a carrier (heterozygous) woman and (B) an affected (hemizygous) man and a normal woman for an X-linked condition.

Table 8-4
Congenital Malformation Recurrence Risk*

	Cleft Lip and/or Cleft Palate	Congenital Dislocation of Hip	Pyloric Stenosis	Talipes Equinovarus	Anencephaly-Meningo-myelocele
Incidence in general population	1/1000	1/1000	2/1000	1/1000	2/1000
Incidence in relatives vs. incidence in general population					
First-degree relatives	35×	40×	20×	20×	8×
Second-degree relatives	7×	4×	5×	5×	—
Third-degree relatives	3×	1.5×	2×	2×	2×

*Increased risk of relatives having the same malformation as a propositus.

163

higher the risk of recurrence. In addition, if the patients with the condition are predominantly of one sex, the risk will be higher to relatives of the less frequently affected sex, who are predisposed to be more extreme deviants.

Analysis of family data has led to the following general conclusions:

1. The etiology of these disorders is multifactorial, involving many different hereditary and environmental influences.
2. The hereditary component is polygenic, i.e., reflecting the activity of many genes and resulting in a continuation of the genetic predisposition.
3. The actual expression requires a strong genetic predisposition that pushes the individual beyond the threshold of risk, at which point environmental influences determine whether and to what extent the patient is affected.

Neural tube defects and prenatal diagnosis.   It is now possible to diagnose neural tube defects by amniocentesis before thg 20th week of gestation. α-Fetoprotein (AFP) is an α-globulin synthesized by embyronal liver cells, the yolk sac, and the fetal gastrointestinal tract. The levels in amniotic fluid rise from the sixth week of embryonic life to a peak at the 14th week and then progressively decrease until birth. However, in the amniotic fluid of a woman carrying a fetus with an open neural tube defect there is an excess of AFP; this makes it possible to screen women with previously affected babies. When the results of amniotic AFP levels, sonography, and x-ray are combined, about 85 percent of neural tube defects can be diagnosed prenatally.

The AFP level in maternal serum also is elevated during the second trimester of pregnancy if the mother is carrying a fetus with an open neural tube defect. If this turns out to be a specific and reliable test, it will then become possible to screen every pregnancy.

CHROMOSOMES

Classification

The diploid number of chromosomes is 46. There are 22 homologous pairs and 2 sex chromosomes. Women have 44 autosomes and 2 X chromosomes (46,XX). Men also have 44 autosomes, but only one X chromosome and one Y chromosome (46,XY). These are classified (Fig. 8–8) on the following bases: (1) length, (2) position of centromere, (3) position of secondary constrictions and presence of satellites, (4) relative rate of replication, and (5) banding patterns.

Homologous pairs of autosomes are numbered 1 to 22 and are divided into seven groups labeled A to G. Within these groups, identification of

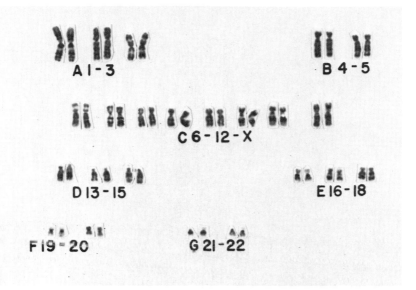

A 1-3

B 4-5

C 6-12-X

D 13-15

E 16-18

F 19-20

G 21-22

Figure 8-8. Karyotype of a normal female showing G banding pattern. Chromosomes are numbered 1–22 (22 pairs plus 2 X chromosomes) and placed into seven groups (A–G).

individual chromosomes can be made by morphologic features (Fig. 8–9) and banding patterns (Figs. 8–10 and 8–11).

The X chromosome is the sixth or seventh longest chromosome. It has a submedian centromere and belongs to group C with autosomes 6 to 12. The Y is similar to the chromosomes in group G (numbers 21 and 22), but it is variable in size, it has shorter short arms that chromosomes 21 and 22, and it does not have satellites.

Chromosomal abnormalities associated with pathologic conditions are the result of alterations in number or structure of chromosomes.

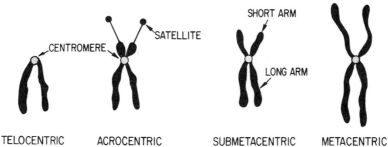

CENTROMERE

SATELLITE

SHORT ARM

LONG ARM

TELOCENTRIC   ACROCENTRIC   SUBMETACENTRIC   METACENTRIC

Figure 8-9. Schematic representation of metaphase chromosomes.

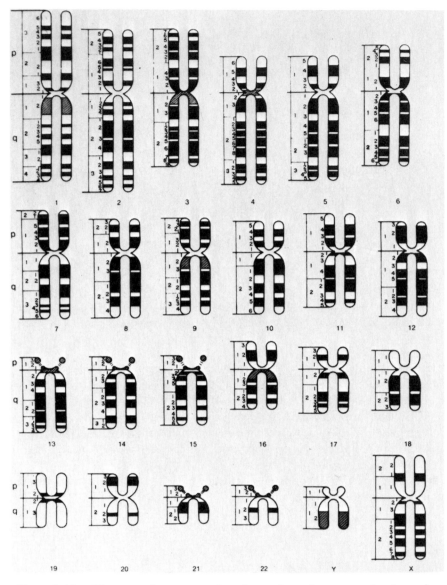

Figure 8-10. Diagrammatic representation of metaphase chromosome bands as observed with Q and G staining methods from the 1971 report of the Paris Conference.

166

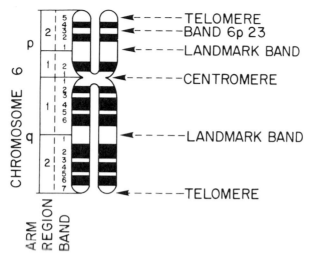

Figure 8-11. Diagrammatic representation of chromosome 6 in metaphase showing details required for identification of any particular band or segment of a chromosome: chromosome number (in this case 6); arm symbol (p = short arm, q = long arm); region and band numbers. For example, 6 p 23 indicates band number 3 of region 2 in the short arm of chromosome 6.

Numerical Alterations (Table 8-5)

For an irregular number of chromosomes, we use the term *aneuploid*. If one of a pair is missing, the number of chromosomes if 45, and we refer to the condition as *monosomy*. If there are three instead of two homologous chromosomes, the number of chromosomes is 47, and we refer to this condition as *trisomy*. Monosomy and trisomy, the most common aneuploids, are caused by meiotic nondisjunction.

MEIOTIC NONDISJUNCTION

When homologous chromosomes fail to separate at anaphase, nondisjunction results. Instead of parting at cell division and each going into a daughter cell, the two chromosomes stick together; thus one daughter cell gets both partners, and the other gets neither. The result is one gamete with 22 chromosomes and one with 24. If the gamete with 22 chromosomes is fertilized by a normal gamete with 23 chromosomes, a zygote with 45 chromosomes (monosomy) is produced. If, on the other hand, the gamete with 24 chromosomes is fertilized by a normal gamete, a zygote with 47 chromosomes (trisomy) is produced. Autosomal and sex chromosome trisomies are common; except for one sex chromosome monosomy (Turner's syndrome), which is relatively common, monosomies are rare.

Table 8–5
Numerical Alterations

Meiotic nondisjunction (NDJ)
  NDJ at first meiotic division
    Autosomal chromosomes:
      Trisomies (47 chromosomes) e.g.:
        Bartholin-Patau syndrome (trisomy 13): 47,XY + 13
        Edward syndrome (trisomy 18): 47,XY + 18
        Down's syndrome (trisomy 21): 47,XY + 21
    Sex chromosomes
      Trisomies (47 chromosomes): Klinefelter's syndrome (47,XXY) and triple X
        syndrome (47,XXX)
      Monosomy (45 chromosomes): Turner's syndrome (45,XO)

  NDJ at second meiotic division, e.g.:
    XYY syndrome (47,XYY)

  NDJ at both meiotic divisions, e.g.:
    48,XXXY
    48,XXXX
    48,XXYY

  Double trisomy (48 chromosomes), e.g.:
    Klinefelter's syndrome and Down's syndrome: 48,XXY + 21

Mitotic nondisjunction (mosaicism), e.g.:
  mos 46,XY/47,XY + 21 (mosaic Down's syndrome)
  mos 46,XX/45,XO (mosaic Turner's syndrome)

Double fertilization: hermaphrodite (chi 46,XX/46,XY)

Polyploidy: common in abortuses, but only few viable cases of triploidy (69
  chromosomes) reported

Trisomy 21.   Trisomy 21 is the most common trisomy syndrome compatible with life; it accounts for 95 percent of all cases of Down's syndrome (Fig. 8–12). The frequency is 1 in about 800 live births. They are virtually all mentally retarded, and at least 30 percent have congenital heart disease, the most common types being ventricular septal defect and endocardial cushion defect (Tables 8–6 and 8–7).

Down's syndrome accounts for 30 percent of retarded children in the United States. The degree of mental retardation varies considerably, but the I.Q. is usually between 40 and 60. Although many patients with Down's

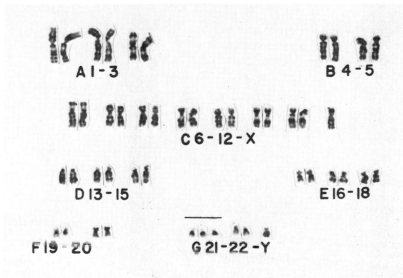

Figure 8-12.   A G-banded karyotype of a boy (XY) with trisomy 21 Down's syndrome. There are 47 chromosomes, the extra one being a number 21 in the G group (47,XY +21).

syndrome have pleasant dispositions, autism and disorders of behavior may be present.

The frequency of acute leukemia in Down's syndrome is about 20 times higher in patients under 15 years of age than in the normal population.

Men with Down's syndrome often have undescended testes; also, libido is diminished, and sperm count is reduced. There are no proven cases of men with Down's syndrome fathering children. In women, secondary sexual characteristics are usually underdeveloped and late in appearing, and menstruation often is absent. Despite this, a small number of women with Down's syndrome have had children; as expected, about half of their children were affected and half were normal, depending on whether or not they received the extra chromosome 21.

About 70 percent of trisomy 21 conceptuses are lost as spontaneous abortions. The life expectancy of a child at birth with Down's syndrome was 9 years in 1929 and 12 years in 1947; it is now better than 20 years. The improved life expectancy is due to improvements in the care of retarded children, cardiac surgery, and the introduction of antibiotics.

Other well-recognized trisomy syndromes are trisomy 13 and trisomy 18 (Tables 8–6 and 8–7).

Table 8–6

Systemic Findings in Some Autosomal Trisomy Syndromes

Bartholin-Patau Syndrome Trisomy D or 13 (47,XX or XY + 13)	Edward Syndrome Trisomy 18 (47,XX or XY + 18)	Down's Syndrome Trisomy 21 (47,XX or XY + 21)
Mental retardation	Mental retardation	Mental retardation
Short stature	Short stature	Short stature
	Hypotonia	Hypotonia
Microcephaly Arhinencephalia Holoprosencephaly	Elongated skull	Brachycephaly Short neck
Micrognathia Cleft lip and palate	Micrognathia Cleft lip and palate Small mouth	Small mouth with protruding tongue
Microphthalmia or anophthalmia		

Low-set, malformed ears
Deafness
	Low-set, malformed ears	Small, low-set,
		    malformed, dysplastic
		    ears

		Flat nasal bridge
	Short sternum	

Polydactyly	Long flexed fingers
	Overlapping fingers
		Short fingers and
		    dysplastic middle
		    phalanx of 5th fingers

Abnormal dermatoglyphics	Abnormal dermatoglyphics	Abnormal dermatoglyphics
	Rockerbottom feet	
		Duodenal atresia and annular pancreas
Undescended testes Renal anomalies		Sterile men
Congenital heart disease	Congenital heart disease VSD and PDA	Congenital heart disease VSD and endocardial cushion defects

Table 8–7
Ocular Findings in Some Autosomal Trisomy Syndromes

Bartholin-Patau Syndrome Trisomy D or 13 (47,XX or XY + 13)	Edward Syndrome Trisomy 18 (47,XX or XY + 18)	Down's Syndrome Trisomy 21 (47,XX or XY + 21)
	Hypoplastic supraorbital ridges	
	Ptosis	
Microphthalmia	Microphthalmia	
	Small oblique palpebral fissures	Mongoloid slant
		Almond-shaped eyes
	Epicanthus	Epicanthus
	Thick lower lid	
	Hypertelorism	Hypotelorism
	Blepharophimosis	Blepharitis
		Strabismus (35%)
		Ectropion
		Myopia
Ciliary and iris coloboma	Uveal coloboma	Brushfield spots (85%)
Cataracts		Cataracts (60%)
Corneal opacities	Corneal opacities	Keratoconus
Persistent hyperplastic primary vitreous		Iris hypoplasia
Intraocular cartilage		Unusual vascular pattern of retina
Rudimentary differentiation of angle structures		
Optic nerve hypoplasia		
Cyclopia		

MITOTIC NONDISJUNCTION

Nondisjunction before fertilization (during meiosis) leads to the production of patients composed entirely of one abnormal chromosome cell line. However, if nondisjunction occurs after fertilization (during mitosis), cells with two or more different chromosome constitutions will result, and hence two or more cell lines will develop.

Patients with mosaic Down's syndrome usually have a 46,XX(or XY)/ 47,XX(or XY) + G karyotype and account for about 2.5 percent of patients with Down's syndrome (Table 8–8). The phenotype of patients with mosaicism varies, as one might expect, from that of a normal person to that typical of a patient with Down's syndrome, depending on proportion and distribution of the trisomic cell line in the body.

Mosaicism may also be found in apparently normal parents of children with Down's syndrome. Fathers of patients with Down's syndrome have been described, all of whom were under 30 years of age, and were mosaics for trisomy 21, as demonstrated in skin, testes, and lymphocytes.

Structural Alterations (Table 8-9)

DELETION

Structural changes are the results of chromosome breaks (Fig. 8–13). If a piece of chromosome breaks off and disappears during cell division because it has no centromere, we are left with a simple deletion. Such deletions have been found in several groups associated with congenital abnormalities (Tables 8–10 and 8–11).

Sometimes pieces of both ends of the same chromosome break off simultaneously and get lost. If the broken ends join with each other, a ring chromosome is formed. Ring chromosome formation of several of the autosomes and X and Y chromosomes also is associated with congenital abnormalities.

An isochromosome is a perfectly metacentric chromosome with two completely homologous arms united at the centromere. It arises by transverse rather than longitudinal splitting at the centromere at the beginning of anaphase. It carries in duplicate the same gene loci of a single chromosome arm that it represents. An isochromosome with a long arm is quite a common structural abnormality of the X chromosome.

TRANSLOCATION

When two breaks occur in different chromosomes, translocation of the detached pieces may occur. Interchanges between either homologous or nonhomologous chromosomes are called reciprocal translocations. Breaks are

Table 8–8
Chromosomal Findings in Down's Syndrome

Abnormal number of chromosomes
  Meiotic nondisjunction
    Trisomy 21: 47,XX + 21 or 47,XY + 21 (95% of cases with Down's
      syndrome)
    Double trisomy
      Down and Klinefelter: 48,XXY + 21 (1:11,000 births)
      Down and triple X: 48,XXX + 21
      Down and XYY: 48,XYY + 21
      Down and trisomy 13
      Down and trisomy 18
  Mitotic nondisjunction (mosaicism)
    47,XX/47,XX + G (2.5% of cases with Down's syndrome)

Abnormal structure of chromosomes
  Translocation syndromes
    Robertsonian translocation (centric fusion): (2.0% of cases with Down's
      syndrome); this process is termed centric fusion because the chromosomes
      rejoin in regions close to the centromeres
    46,XX,t(13q21q) or 46,XY,t(13q21q) (very rare)
    46,XX,t(14q21q) or 46,XY,t(14q21q) (unusual type)
    46,XX,t(15q21q) or 46,XY,t(15q21q) (rare)
    46,XX,t(21q22q) or 46,XY,t(21q22q)
    46,XX,t(21q21) or 46,XY,t(21q21)
    46,XX,t(21qi) (isochromosome of long arms of No. 21)
    46,XX,tan(21q21q) (tandem of long arms of No. 21)
  Translocations also have been described that result in Down's syndrome:
    Between No. 1 and No. 21
    Between No. 2 and No. 21
    Between No. 6 and No. 21
    Between No. 7 and No. 21
    Between No. 19 and No. 21
  Reciprocal translocations (partial trisomy): 47,XY or XX, 21q−
                                                47,XY or XX,21p−
  Trisomy of the distal portion of the long arm of chromosome 21 is necessary for
  the phenotypic features of Down's syndrome. Gradations of clinical features in
  the syndrome are due to loss of varying amounts distally from the long arms of a
  21 chromosome; consequently, trisomy of the most distal segment may be
  pathogenetic in the syndrome.

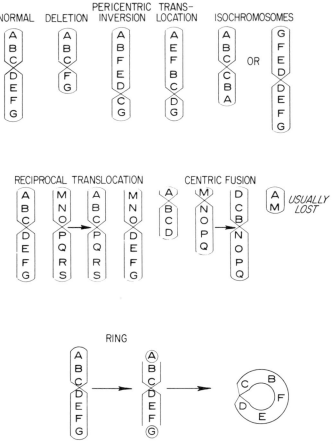

Figure 8-13. Diagrammatic representation of various forms of structural alterations of chromosomes.

assumed to take place at or near the centromere of the two nonhomologous chromosomes and to be followed by a translocation and rejoining. This process is called centric fusion because the chromosomes rejoin in regions close to the centromere. The result of reciprocal translocation is loss of chromosome material and alteration of chromosome structure. If a gamete in which a reciprocal translocation is present becomes fertilized by a normal gamete, zygotes with normal as well as balanced chromosomal constitutions may result. A zygote with a balanced chromosomal constitution develops into a phenotypically normal person. Such people will, however, run a considerable risk of having miscarriages and children with congenital abnormalities as a result of producing zygotes with unbalanced chromosomal constitution. The important point is that translocation chromosomes can be inherited through

Table 8–9

Structural Alterations

Deletion syndromes
 Simple deletions, e.g.:
  Group B: Short-arm deletion of 4 (Wolf-Hirschhorn syndrome, 4−)
       Short-arm deletion of 5 (cri du chat syndrome, 5p−)
  Group E: Short- and long-arm deletions of 18 (18p− and 18q−)
  Group G: Long-arm deletion of chromosome 21
       21 (G deletion syndrome I, antimongolism, 21q−)
       22 (G deletion syndrome II, 22q−)
  X chromosome: short- and long-arm deletions (46,XXp− and 46,XXq−)
  Double deletions (ring chromosome formation): 46, r(X)
  Deletions caused by misdivision (isochromosomes):
   Long-arm isochromosome = short-arm deletion: 46,X, i(Xq)
   Short-arm isochromosome = long-arm deletion: 46,X, i(Xp)

Translocation syndromes
 Robertsonian translocation (centric fusion), e.g.:
  D/G (14/21) translocation Down's syndrome: 46,XX (or XY), D−,t(DqGq)+
 Reciprocal translocations (partial trisomy), e.g.:
  22q+ (cat's eye syndrome)

---

phenotypically normal carriers (see Table 8–13). There are two types of translocation Down's syndrome (Table 8–8):

Patients with 46,XX(or XY), G−,t(DqGq) + karyotype of translocation Down's syndrome are phenotypically indistinguishable from those with trisomy 21 (Fig. 8–14). The abnormality may be inherited from a phenotypically normal parent who carries the translocation chromosome.

Patients with 46XX(or XY), G−,t(GqGq) + karyotype account for slightly more than the 1 percent of patients with Down's syndrome (Fig. 8–15). There are two varieties of this translocation (21/21 and 21/22 centric fusion); they also account for some examples of familial Down's syndrome.

The chance of having a child with trisomy 21 increases with advancing maternal age (Table 8–12). Now that it is possible to examine the chromosomes of fetal cells obtained by amniocentesis, pregnant women over the age of 35 should be offered the opportunity of prenatal diagnosis. This also should be offered to women who have had a previous child with Down's syndrome and when one of the parents is known to be a translocation carrier (Table 8–13).

Chromosomal anomalies of the type involving number 21 also involve many of the others, and these also are associated with malformation syndromes, many of which are severe and lead to miscarriages. The frequency of chromosomal abnormalities in spontaneous abortuses is about 20 percent.

Table 8–10
Systemic Findings in Some Autosomal Deletion Syndromes

Wolf-Hirschhorn Syndrome Short-Arm Deletion of Chromosome 4 (46,XX or XY, 4p−)	Cri du Chat Syndrome Short-Arm Deletion of Chromosome 5 (46,XX or XY, 5p−)	Long-Arm Deletion of Chromosome 13 (46,XX or XY, 13q−)	De Grouchy Syndrome Long-Arm Deletion of Chromosome 18 (46,XX or XY, 18q−)	G Deletion Syndrome II Long-Arm Deletion of Chromosome 21 (46,XX or XY, 21q−)
Mental retardation	Mental retardation	Mental retardation	Mental retardation	Mental retardation
	Catlike cry			
Short stature	Short stature	Short stature	Short stature	Short stature
Hypotonia	Hypotonia			Hypotonia
Microcephaly	Microcephaly	Microcephaly	Microcephaly	Microcephaly
Midline defects	Moonface	Holoprosencephaly	Hypoplastic maxilla	
Micrognathia	Micrognathia			
Carp mouth		Protruding upper incisors	Carp mouth	
Cleft palate				
Eye defects (Table 8–11)	Eye defects (Table 8–11)	Eye defects (Table 8–11)	Eye defects (Table 8–11)	Antimongoloid slant to palpebral fissure

Table 8–10 (*continued*)
Systemic Findings in Some Autosomal Deletion Syndromes

Wolf-Hirschhorn Syndrome Short-Arm Deletion of Chromosome 4 (46,XX or XY, 4p−)	Cri du Chat Syndrome Short-Arm Deletion of Chromosome 5 (46,XX or XY, 5p−)	Long-Arm Deletion of Chromosome 13 (46,XX or XY, 13q−)	De Grouchy Syndrome Long-Arm Deletion of Chromosome 18 (46,XX or XY, 18q−)	G Deletion Syndrome II Long-Arm Deletion of Chromosome 21 (46,XX or XY, 21q−)
Low-set ears	Low-set ears	Ear anomalies	Prominent anthelix and tragus	Large, low-set ears
Periauricular dimple			Atretic external ear canal	
			Conductive hearing loss	
Beaked nose				
Broad nasal bridge	Broad nasal bridge	Broad nasal bridge		Prominent nasal bridge
Simian creases	Syndactyly	Hypoplastic or absent thumbs		Nail anomalies
	Simian creases	Long fingers	Simian crease	
Foot deformities	Foot deformities	Vertebral agenesis		Skeletal anomalies
		Dislocated hips		
Undescended testes	Undescended testes	Genitourinary anomalies	Genitourinary anomalies	Pyloric stenosis
Hypospadias				Hypospadias and cryptorchidism
Congenital heart disease	Congenital heart disease	Congenital heart disease	Congenital heart disease	

Table 8-11
Ocular Findings in Some Autosomal Deletion Syndromes

Wolf-Hirschhorn Syndrome Short-Arm Deletion of Chromosome 4 (46,XX or XY, 4p−)	Cri du Chat Syndrome Short-Arm Deletion of Chromosome 5 (46,XX or XY, 5p−)	Long-Arm Deletion of Chromosome 13 (46,XX or XY, 13q−)	De Grouchy Syndrome Long-Arm Deletion of Chromosome 18 (46,XX or XY, 18q−)
Defect of eyebrows	Absence of eyebrows		
Antimongoloid slant	Antimongoloid slant		
Hypertelorism	Hypertelorism	Hypertelorism	Hypertelorism
Ptosis		Ptosis	Ptosis
	Epicanthus	Epicanthus	Epicanthus
Exophthalmos	Microphthalmia	Microphthalmia	Microphthalmia
			Microcornea
			Corneal opacity
Exotropia	Exotropia		Strabismus
	Strabismus		
	Blepharoptosis		
	Telecanthus		
Coloboma	Coloboma	Coloboma	Coloboma
	Cataract	Cataract	Myopia
	Hypertropia	Retinoblastoma	Glaucoma
	Amblyopia		Muscular abnormalities
	Ocular dermoid		
	Optic atrophy		Optic atrophy
	Tortuous retinal vessels		

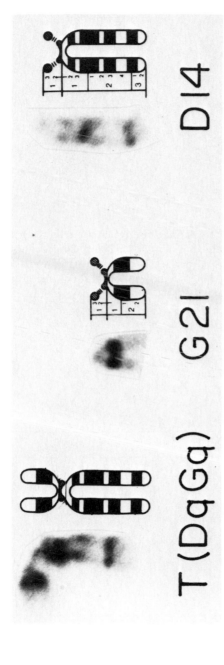

Figure 8-14. Morphology and G banding of a D/G translocation chromosome resulting from the transfer of the long arms (q) of a number 21 chromosome from group G onto the long arms (q) of a number 14 chromosome from group D. This was obtained from a boy with Down's syndrome who had the following karyotype: 46,XY, G−,t(DqGq)+.

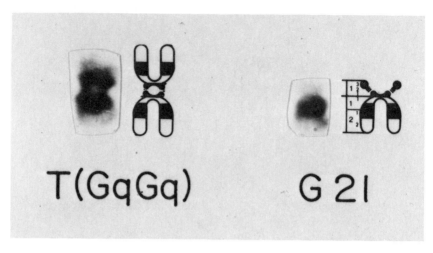

Figure 8-15.   Morphology and G banding of a G/G translocation chromosome resulting from the transfer of the long arms (q) of a number 21 chromosome from group G onto the long arms (q) of another number 21 chromosome from group G. This was obtained from a girl with Down's syndrome who had the following karyotype: 46,XX, G−,t(GqGq)+.

Table 8–12
Down's Syndrome and Maternal Age*

Maternal Age (years)	Risk
<30	1:1500
30–34	1:750
34	1:527
35	1:413
36	1:333
37	1:266
38	1:183
39	1:135
40	1:108
41	1:83

*The general risk of having a child with Down's syndrome is related to the mother's age. About 1–5% of mothers are over the age of 40 years, and they contribute 16% of cases of Down's syndrome. Mothers 35 years of age and over contribute about 35% of cases.

Table 8–13
Genetic Prognosis

Patient	Mother	Father	Recurrence Risk
Trisomy 21	Normal	Normal	Maternal-age-dependent
D:21 translocation	Normal	Normal	Small
D:21 translocation	Carrier	Normal	1:9
21:21 translocation	Normal	Normal	Small
21:21 translocation	Carrier	Normal	100%
21:21 translocation	Normal	Carrier	100%
21:22 translocation	Normal	Normal	Small
21:22 translocation	Carrier	Normal	1:8–1:10
21:22 translocation	Normal	Carrier	1:8–1:10
Mosaic	Normal	Normal	1%
	Mosaic	Normal	10–15%
	Trisomy 21	Normal	50%
	Normal	Trisomy 21	50%

The classic trisomy syndrome involving the sex chromosomes is Klinefelter's syndrome (48,XXY) (Table 8–5), a condition characterized by eunuchoid body proportions, gynecomastia, small testes, and aspermia. The classic monosomy syndrome involving the sex chromosomes is Turner's syndrome (45,X) (Table 8–5), a condition having as its cardinal features short stature, infantilism, streak gonads, and a number of eye (Table 8–14) and other congenital anomalies.

Mosaicism and structural chromosomal anomalies are common in Turner's syndrome and related conditions. Chromosomal studies also are invaluable in patients with ambiguous external genitalia.

Chromosomes and Malignancy

Most patients with bilateral retinoblastoma have normal chromosomes, and the condition is inherited as an autosomal dominant with incomplete penetrance. However, the association of a deletion of chromosome 13 in a few patients with retinoblastoma is of considerable interest. The chromosome anomaly is present in all body cells examined, and the patients vary from almost normal to severely malformed infants.

The best-known association between a chromosomal anomaly and malignancy is the presence of the so-called Philadelphia chromosome (Ph[1]) in 90 percent of patients with chronic myeloid leukemia. Patients with this form of leukemia and the Ph[1] chromosome have a better prognosis than those without the chromosomal anomaly. The Ph[1] is usually a 22/9 translocation.

Table 8–14
Ocular Findings in Turner's Syndrome

Prominent epicanthal folds
Ptosis
Strabismus
Pigmented areas on lids
Incidence of color blindness same as in men
Eccentric pupil
Cataract

Study of the association of chromosomal anomalies in malignancy is a field of rapidly growing interest and importance.

REFERENCES

1. Goldberg MF (ed): Genetic and Metabolic Eye Diseases. Boston, Little, Brown, 1974.
2. McKusick VA: Mendelian Inheritance in Man (ed. 4). Baltimore, Johns Hopkins University Press, 1975.
3. Ophthalmology. Basic and Clinical Science course. Section 2. Anatomy, Embryology, Genetics and Developmental Abnormalities. November-December, 1976. American Academy of Ophthalmology and Otolaryngology. p 131
4. Smith DA: Recognizable Patterns of Human Malformation (ed 2). Philadelphia, WB Saunders, 1976.
5. Sorsby A: Ophthalmic Genetics (ed 2). New York, Appleton-Century-Crofts, 1970.
6. Stevenson AC, Davison BCC, Oakes MW: Genetic Counseling (ed 2). Philadelphia, JB Lippincott, 1976.
7. Warburg M: Diagnosis of Metabolic Eye Diseases. Copenhagen, Munksgaard, 1972.
8. Yunis JJ (ed): New Chromosomal Syndromes. New York, Academic Press, 1977.

Index